AF686436

THE SQUIBB INSTITUTE FOR MEDICAL RESEARCH
LIBRARY
SEP 14 1984
PRINCETON, N. J.

DISCARD

Radionuclide Generators

ACS SYMPOSIUM SERIES 241

Radionuclide Generators

New Systems for Nuclear Medicine Applications

Furn F. Knapp, Jr., EDITOR
Thomas A. Butler, EDITOR
Oak Ridge National Laboratory

Based on a symposium sponsored by
the Division of Nuclear Chemistry and Technology
at the 185th Meeting
of the American Chemical Society,
Seattle, Washington,
March 20–25, 1983

American Chemical Society, Washington, D.C. 1984

Library of Congress Cataloging in Publication Data

Radionuclide generators.

(ACS symposium series, ISSN 0097-6156; 241)

"Based on a symposium sponsored by the Division of Nuclear Chemistry and Technology at the 185th Meeting of the American Chemical Society, Seattle, Washington, March 20-25, 1983."

1. Nuclear medicine—Congresses. 2. Radionuclide generators—Congresses. I. Knapp, F. F., 1944- . II. Butler, Thomas A. (Thomas Arthur), 1919- . III. American Chemical Society. Division of Nuclear Chemistry and Technology. IV. American Chemical Society Meeting (185th: 1983: Seattle, Wash.) V. Series. [DNLM: 1. Radionuclide generators—Instrumentation—Congresses. 2. Radioisotopes—Congresses. WN 150]

R895.A2R33 1984 616.07'57 83-25875
ISBN 0-8412-0822-0

Copyright © 1984

American Chemical Society

All Rights Reserved. The appearance of the code at the bottom of the first page of each chapter in this volume indicates the copyright owner's consent that reprographic copies of the chapter may be made for personal or internal use or for the personal or internal use of specific clients. This consent is given on the condition, however, that the copier pay the stated per copy fee through the Copyright Clearance Center, Inc. for copying beyond that permitted by Sections 107 or 108 of the U.S. Copyright Law. This consent does not extend to copying or transmission by any means—graphic or electronic—for any other purpose, such as for general distribution, for advertising or promotional purposes, for creating a new collective work, for resale, or for information storage and retrieval systems. The copying fee for each chapter is indicated in the code at the bottom of the first page of the chapter.

The citation of trade names and/or names of manufacturers in this publication is not to be construed as an endorsement or as approval by ACS of the commercial products or services referenced herein; nor should the mere reference herein to any drawing, specification, chemical process, or other data be regarded as a license or as a conveyance of any right or permission, to the holder, reader, or any other person or corporation, to manufacture, reproduce, use, or sell any patented invention or copyrighted work that may in any way be related thereto. Registered names, trademarks, etc., used in this publication, even without specific indication thereof, are not to be considered unprotected by law.

PRINTED IN THE UNITED STATES OF AMERICA

ACS Symposium Series

M. Joan Comstock, *Series Editor*

Advisory Board

Robert Baker
U.S. Geological Survey

Martin L. Gorbaty
Exxon Research and Engineering Co.

Herbert D. Kaesz
University of California—Los Angeles

Rudolph J. Marcus
Office of Naval Research

Marvin Margoshes
Technicon Instruments Corporation

Donald E. Moreland
USDA, Agricultural Research Service

W. H. Norton
J. T. Baker Chemical Company

Robert Ory
USDA, Southern Regional Research Center

Geoffrey D. Parfitt
Carnegie-Mellon University

Theodore Provder
Glidden Coatings and Resins

James C. Randall
Phillips Petroleum Company

Charles N. Satterfield
Massachusetts Institute of Technology

Dennis Schuetzle
Ford Motor Company Research Laboratory

Davis L. Temple, Jr.
Mead Johnson

Charles S. Tuesday
General Motors Research Laboratory

C. Grant Willson
IBM Research Department

FOREWORD

The ACS SYMPOSIUM SERIES was founded in 1974 to provide a medium for publishing symposia quickly in book form. The format of the Series parallels that of the continuing ADVANCES IN CHEMISTRY SERIES except that in order to save time the papers are not typeset but are reproduced as they are submitted by the authors in camera-ready form. Papers are reviewed under the supervision of the Editors with the assistance of the Series Advisory Board and are selected to maintain the integrity of the symposia; however, verbatim reproductions of previously published papers are not accepted. Both reviews and reports of research are acceptable since symposia may embrace both types of presentation.

CONTENTS

PREFACE

THE DEVELOPMENT OF CLINICAL RADIONUCLIDE GENERATORS has been a significant factor contributing to the rapid growth of nuclear medicine practice. Technetium-99m obtained from the Mo-99/Tc-99m generator system is the most widely used radionuclide for in vivo diagnostic tests. The purpose of the symposium on new radionuclide generator systems for nuclear medicine was to review the state of development of new radionuclide generator systems for application in both diagnostic and therapeutic nuclear medicine. The program was broadly divided into three sessions on short-lived radionuclides, positron-emitting radionuclides, and radionuclide production and miscellaneous applications.

Interest in new generator-derived single photon-emitting radionuclides has increased in recent years due in part to advances in "fast" gamma cameras that allow very high count rates and computerized image reconstruction techniques. In addition, use of short-lived radionuclides such as Au-195m (30.5 sec), Ir-191m (5 sec), Kr-81 (13.3 sec), and Ta-178 (9.3 min) for radionuclide angiography allows repeat studies at short intervals with significant reduction in absorbed radiation dose; thus, therapeutic intervention can be assessed. This is particularly important in pediatric applications, such as the evaluation of intracardiac shunts in children with Ir-191m.

The wide availability of positron emission tomographic instrumentation has stimulated the use of generator-derived positron-emitting radionuclides such as Rb-82, Mn-52m, and Ga-68. The availability of these generator-derived radionuclides is very important for positron tomography studies and now allows use of the procedure at facilities which are remote from production sites. The on-site cyclotron is no longer essential for patient examination by positron tomography. Radionuclides with therapeutic applications, such as the alpha emitter Bi-212, can also be obtained from radionuclide generators and are of interest for attachment to tissue-specific monoclonal antibodies.

All of the above radionuclides obtained from generator systems were discussed in this symposium. The symposium offered a good opportunity to review and discuss in detail the new generation and improved versions of older radionuclide generators that are being developed for nuclear medicine applications. Our goal at this symposium was to emphasize the chemical and mechanical aspects of generator design and performance. We were pleased to have representatives from the private sector participate and describe advances in radionuclide generator systems that will be commercially available to provide the medical community a ready access to important new diagnostic aids. The chapters in this volume also review the clinical applications of these generators to provide a comprehensive overview of generator design, development, and use. We felt there was a real need for a book describing the recent developments in radionuclide generators. This book will be of interest to basic researchers, clinicians, technicians, and other professionals working in the nuclear medicine area.

We would like to express our thanks to all of our colleagues who participated in this symposium, including Thomas F. Budinger who took time from his busy schedule to present the keynote address. We also thank Linda Ailey for her enthusiasm and help in coordinating the manuscript correspondence and those who reviewed the manuscripts to help make this important volume available to the scientific community.

FURN F. KNAPP, JR.
THOMAS A. BUTLER
Oak Ridge National Laboratory
Oak Ridge, Tennessee

August 1983

SHORT-LIVED RADIONUCLIDES

1

A New Generator for Production of Short-Lived Au-195m Radioisotope

K. J. PANEK, J. LINDEYER, and H. C. VAN DER VLUGT

Byk-Mallinckrodt CIL B.V., Cyclotron & Isotope Laboratories, P.O. Box 3, 1755 ZG Petten, Holland

A generator has been developed to produce multimillicurie amounts of 30.6 second Au-195m. Gold-195m, a daughter isotope of 41.6 hour Hg-195m, is eluted as neutral and sterile sodium thiosulphatoaurate(I) complex, and as such, is indicated for dynamic studies in cardiology. Mercury-195m is produced by irradiation of gold targets with 28 MeV protons, yielding by the (p,3n) nuclear reaction Hg-195m and Hg-195 (9.9 hours) at rates of 4.6 and 12 mCi/μAh, respectively. Mercury is separated from irradiated gold by distillation and collection in nitric acid. This solution is neutralized and loaded on a column of silica gel modified with metallic sulphide. Columns are eluted at 3-5 minute intervals with a solution containing 29.8 mg/ml sodium thiosulphate, pentahydrate and 10 mg/ml sodium nitrate. Yields of Au-195m vary between 24-45% of theory, depending on the total Hg activity and the generator production method. Gold-195m is obtained in 3-4 seconds by eluting with 2 ml under pressure. Contamination of the eluate with mercury isotopes decreases after about 20 elutions to 0.4 - 0.8 μCi Hg-195m/mCi Au-195m.

Although the Os-191/Ir-191m system is one of the potentially interesting generators for the ultra short-lived radionuclides (USLR) and was described by Campbell and Nelson (1) as early as in 1956, it was only the growing interest for application of USLR in cardiology, that stimulated a broader research in this field. As a result, a number of generators like Cd-109/Ag-109m (2), Os-191/Ir-191m (2, 3), Rb-81/Kr-81m (4), Br-77/Se-77m (5), W-178/Ta-178 (6) have been studied in the last years. The Hg-195m/Au-195m generator was theoretically considered by Lebowitz (7) and experimentally studied by Yano (8), apparently

0097-6156/84/0241-0003$06.00/0
© 1984 American Chemical Society

without successful conclusion. From the published data on the existing generator systems, it was however seen, that none of the USLR obtained from these generators was optimum for the intended application in cardiology (Table I). In addition, none of the generator systems (except for Kr-81m) worked efficiently and economically and none were suitable for larger scale or commercial production.

Evaluating the advantages and disadvantages of the three potentially most promising candidates for USLR generators, i.e. Cd-109/Ag-109m, Os-191/Ir-191m and Hg-195m/Au-195m (Table II), we came to the conclusion that the latter parent-daughter pair represents the best possible compromise.

Table I. Generators for USLR - Specification of Isotopes

Parent Isotope :	$T_{1/2}$ long enough for transportation Photon energy not too high, permitting effective shielding High decay yield to daughter isotope
Daughter Isotope:	$T_{1/2}$ optimally ca 20 sec. Photon energy between 80 - 250 keV High photon emission yield Chemical form that stays in the circulation

Table II. Potential candidates for USLR Generators

	Advantage	Disadvantage
Os-191/Ir-191m	$T_{1/2}$ Parent Reactor isotope Photon energy daughter	Parent beta emitter Loading mg quantities per generator $T_{1/2}$ daughter too short Low photon yield Iridium chemistry
Cd-109/Ag-109m	$T_{1/2}$ Daughter Photon energy daughter	$T_{1/2}$ Parent too long Low production rate Low photon yield
Hg-195m/Au-195m	$T_{1/2}$ Daughter High photon yield Acceptable production rate Carrier free parent isotope	$T_{1/2}$ Parent somewhat short

Theoretical considerations. By the nature of the intended application of Au-195m, requiring direct linking of the generator to the patient, it was obvious that the separation system and generator design must possess a number of specific features, as for instance given in Table III. These requirements had a direct technical consequences for the separation chemistry and selection of materials for the generator construction. For instance, a small column containing minimal bed material would limit the maximum amount of parent isotope that could be loaded to only a few milligrams. Inorganic sorbents, preferable for their radiation stability, usually have lower adsorption capacity and might even require loading with carrier-free parent isotope. A short column bed together with the expected large number of successive elutions would require extremely good fixation of the parent isotope to the column bed to make it virtually non elutable. To design a purposeful, yet not too excessive experimental scheme, we decided to focus our research on inorganic sorbents. To acquire in a short time as much information as possible, we further decided to divide the problem of the generator (adsorption of the parent isotope and elution of daughter), and to investigate the adsorption of mercury and gold separately. Since we expected that for each particular sorbent a "matching" eluent would have to be found, the above mentioned division of the adsorption-elution problem made it possible to screen rapidly (in batch adsorption experiments) a large number of sorbent-eluent combinations, which would be otherwise impossible to test in column experiments.

Because of the vast variety of known sorbents useable for adsorption of mercury, it was clear that the screening experiments could not be exhaustive, but should be at least representative for the potentially useful groups of sorbents with related properties. Thus we included sorbents from the group of hydrated oxides silica gel, hydrated manganese dioxide (HMDO), hydrated zirconium oxide and alumina, phosphates (zirconium phosphate) and as a generally useful sorbent charcoal was also added. To exploit the affinity of mercury to sulphur and its compounds, sorbents containing elemental sulphur and metallic sulphides (silver sulphide and zinc sulphide) were also included. To test at least some of the recently developed, and potentially very useful sorbents from the group of anchored chelates, two representative sorbents were chosen, silica gel with chemically bonded mercaptopropyl groups (SiO_2-SH), which exploits the affinity to sulphur, and silica gel with chemically bonded aminopropyl groups (SiO_2-NH_2), exploiting the affinity of mercury to amines. As a last group we tested sorbents coated with metals. These were represented by Ag coated SiO_2 and Au coated SiO_2. Since some of the selected materials (sulphur, zinc sulphide, etc) were not mechanically suitable (fine powders) it was decided to use such materials in a form of modified sorbents, i.e. mechanically suitable carrier material (silica gel) coated with the active sorbent in question.

Table III. Specifications of Separation System for USLR

Sorbent	:	Material stable against radiation, preferably inorganic Nontoxic Insoluble Good mechanical properties Good packing and flow characteristics (of the column) Easy to prepare and handle Very strong binding of parent isotope, preferably total immobilization
Eluent	:	Nonreactive towards adsorbed parent isotope Rapidly reacting with daughter isotope Converting daughter isotope to chemical form nonreactive to sorbent Nontoxic Physiological pH Isotonic Chemically stable
Eluate	:	Obtained in low volume ≤2 ml With high elution yield Minimum breakthrough of parent isotope in large number of elutions Sterile Pyrogen-free
Generator system	:	Small columns, <1 ml void Radiation resistant materials Nonadsorbing either parent or daughter isotope High loading - up to 1000 mCi/generator Adequate shielding Simple and fast production Simple operation System allowing direct connection to patient

Experimental

Adsorption of mercury. All chemicals used were Merck or Baker analytical quality reagents, unless stated otherwise. From the commercially available adsorbents the following were used: silica gel 60 A^{o} porosity, 0.063-0.200 mm particle size (Merck); charcoal 0.3-0.5 mm particle size, gas-chromatographic quality (Merck); alumina R Woelm; hydrous zirconium oxide HZO-1, 100-200 mesh, (Bio-Rad). Except for zirconium phosphate, which was prepared according to Amphlett (9), all other sorbents were prepared by coating (precipitation) on acid-purified silica gel, as described in (10). The SiO_2-NH_2 was prepared according to Leyden et al (11).

Batch adsorption experiments. All experiments were performed with Hg-203 (TRC Amersham), to determine the distribution coefficient K_D defined as:

$$K_D = (\frac{A_0}{A_1} - 1) \times \frac{\text{ml aqueous phase}}{\text{g sorbent}} = X \text{ ml/g}$$

where A_0 is the count rate of the original solution, and A_1 is the count rate of solution (supernatant) after equilibration with the sorbent.

For a typical batch adsorption experiment 500 mg of the dry sorbent and 5.0 ml of liquid phase formulated to the desired (constant) composition and pH were sealed in acid prewashed 10 ml screw cap vials with teflon closures and shaken for 18 hours. After shaking, the vials were centrifuged to remove the fines from the supernatant and an aliquot of the supernatant was counted against a standard of the particular formulated liquid phase. All experiments were performed in triplicate, at constant activity and Hg-carrier concentration (20 μg Hg/ml) with controls (liquid phase without sorbent) to check for possible adsorption losses on the container. The experiments were carried out in nitrate and chloride media at pH 1-10.

Results of batch adsorption experiments. The observed K_D values varied widely for different sorbents and acid concentrations, being as low as ~1 for SiO_2-sulphur and as high as 10^5 for charcoal. Although K_D, as defined above, is not directly translatable to dynamic (loading of the generator columns) experiments, where also the capacity and particularly adsorption rate are very important, still one can presume that sorbents with K_D <10^2 are (as column beds) practically useless. Sorbents with K_D 10^2-10^3, when used as column bed, would probably retain a large part of activity during loading, but there is a danger of larger breakthrough of the adsorbed activity in the following treatment (washing, elutions), particularly when the composition of the liquid phase is changed. Only sorbents with K_D >10^3 could be expected to make a good column bed with relatively small breakthrough, supposing that their adsorption capacity is well above the amount of the loaded element. The sorbents found to fulfil this K_D requirement are shown in Table IV. The fact that the highest K_D values were found at pH 4-6 also indicated what conditions should have been used for loading of a generator column. Although the results obtained in experiments with chloride systems were almost identical to those obtained with nitrates, the latter system is preferable because of lower volatility of mercury.

Table IV. Adsorption of Mercury(Hg-203)in Nitrate System,K_D($x10^3$)

pH	Adsorption agent	SiO_2 HMDO	SiO_2 ZnS	SiO_2 Ag_2S	SiO_2 Ag	C	SiO_2 -SH	SiO_2 $-NH_2$
3		0.016	4.6	11	6.4	55	2.2	2.8
4		4.2	5.3	23	5.8	580	2.5	2.7
5		4.2	2.2	13	3.8	110	2.2	3.1
6		4.4	4.3	4.0	2.0	16	2.5	3.3
7		4.7	3.2	5.1	0.95	130	3.1	3.5
8		4.3	0.033	1.3	0.50	100	1.8	3.5

Adsorption of gold complexes. In principle it was expected that gold in a simple chemical form, like e.g. sodium tetrachloroaurate, would probably be adsorbed on the selected sorbents as strongly as mercury because of the similar properties of both elements and would therefore not be easily "elutable". This raised the question as to what chemical form would make gold nonreactive toward the sorbents, without affecting the adsorbed mercury. The selection of possible compounds to be tested was to a large extent limited by requirements such as low toxicity, pharmaceutical acceptability, solubility, rapid formation of the gold complex (in situ) at the desired pH, and good stability.

Since it was clear that the number of gold complexing agents to be tested could not be exhaustive, we concentrated on organic amines ant thiols or combinations thereof. This choice was motivated by possible competition for gold between sorbent and eluent when both contained the same active groups (bonded phases). As a third group, simple inorganic complexing agents with known high affinities for gold (bromide, thiosulphate and rhodanide) were also investigated.

Batch adsorption experiments. The complexing agents tested were of following origin: mercaptosuccinic acid (TM) - Baker; glutathione, reduced (GTT) - Calbiochem, A grade; α-mercaptopropionylglycine (MPG) - Calbiochem, A grade; thiosalicylic acid (TS) puriss. - Fluka; mercaptoacetic acid (TG) - Baker; L(+) arginine (ARG) - Baker; p-amino hippuric acid (PAH) - Baker; L-threonine (THR) - Merck; tris (hydroxymethyl) amino-methane (TRIS) - Baker. AR grade; sodium thiosulphate (THIO) - Merck, AR grade. Sodium bromide (BR) and sodium thiocyanate (SCN) as well as all other chemicals were Baker, AR grade.

Gold complexes, labelled with Au-198, were prepared from the compounds described above and tested in combination with sorbents identified in Table IV. A similar experimental scheme with one modification was used as for the experiments with mercury. To simulate the "generator" conditions as closely as possible (neutral eluent and carrier-free Au) the tests were performed only at pH 5-6 and with the lowest technically possible concentration of Au carrier (1 μg/ml). Conditions for each experiment were the following: solid phase 500 mg, liquid phase 5 ml, shaking time 18 hours, and sampling of supernatant and counting as for mercury adsorption experiments. The liquid phase (solutions of the Au-198 complexes) was prepared from (Au-198) $HAuCl_4$ and an excess of the complexing agent (usually a 10 mM solution) and brought to a pH of 5. After dilution with water the solutions had the following composition: complexing agent concentration, 1 mM; Au, 1 μg/ml; activity, 1-2 μCi Au-198/ml, pH 5-6. All tests were carried out in triplicate.

From the interpretation of the values K_D with respect to "elution yield" can be derived that for a good "elution yield" (≥70%) a combination with K_D 0.1-5 would be needed. Complexing agents meeting this criterion, namely THIO, TRIS, PAH, GTT, MPG and TM were further tested in column experiments.

Column experiments. These experiments were aimed at two objectives. First, to verify the suitability of those sorbent/complex combinations, identified in batch adsorption experiments, for column operation, particularly with respect to the possible breakthrough of Hg-203, and, second, to study the effect of the concentration of complexing agent on the "elution characteristics" of a generator column. For both groups of experiments we used small glass columns (6.5 mm I.D.) packed with 500 mg of the particular sorbents, prewashed with 5 ml 1 mM nitrate solution pH 5-6 and loaded with Hg-203 solution (20 μg Hg/ml of 1 mM nitrate, pH 5-6). The loaded columns were once more washed with 3 ml of nitrate solution and eluted with 50 ml of Au-complex solution. The column effluents were collected in 5 ml fractions and counted against the standard sample of Hg-203 loading solution to determine the Hg-breakthrough percentage. It was found that only SiO_2-ZnS, SiO_2-SH and SiO_2-NH_2 showed the best properties with no detectable breakthrough for a number of Au-complexes. The SiO_2-Ag showed a small breakthrough (≤0.1%) with all of the Au-complexes; SiO_2-Ag_2S gave no detectable breakthrough only with Au-THIO and SiO_2-HMDO gave no detectable breakthrough only with Au-TRIS and Au-PAH.

In the second group of experiments, using the same experimental technique, the Hg-203 loaded columns were eluted with solutions of Au-198-complexes with constant Au-198 activity and carrier concentration (1 μg Au/ml), but with varying concentration of the Au-complexing agent (0.001-0.1 M) to study the effect of the complexing agent concentration on the simulated "elution yield". It was found that in almost all tested combinations the simulated "elution yield" was concentration dependent, as for example seen in Figure 1 for the SiO_2-ZnS/THIO combination. The overview of the best results obtained for the simulated "elution yield" (% of recovery of Au-198-complexes) are summarized in Table V. Taking into account these results in combination with other aspects such as the ease of the preparation of the particular sorbent, properties and stability of the gold-complexing agent solutions (eluent) and the stability of Au-complexes (eluate), the best choice for generator development seemed to be SiO_2-ZnS/THIO. As an active component of the sorbent, ZnS showed in this system only low affinity to Au-THIO complex, and THIO did not cause a breakthrough of the adsorbed mercury. Both SiO_2-NH_2 and particularly SiO_2-SH were very good and also quite intriguing sorbents. The latter is functionally almost identical to a sorbent used in another Hg-195m/Au-195m generator system, that was developed by Bett et al (12-14). Their generator, however, must be eluted with a solution of sodium cyanide to obtain a reasonable elution yield of Au-195m. We have performed

Table V. Overview of Column Experiments Simulating the "Elution yield" of Au-198-complexes*.

Combination	THIO	TRIS	PAH	GTT	MPG	TM
SiO_2-HMDO		0.1 90%	0.1 > 50%			
SiO_2-ZnS	0.1 97%					
SiO_2-Ag_2S				0.005 85%		0.005 60%
SiO_2-Ag				0.01 95%	0.01 95%	0.01 95%
SiO_2SH	0.1 70%	0.1 18%	0.1 1-5%			
SiO_2-NH_2		0.1 80%				

* For each combination the top figure = molarity of complexing agent, lower figure = percentage of Au-198 activity recovered in eluate.

a number of experiments with this excellent sorbent (SiO_2-SH) in an attempt to modify its very strong affinity to noncomplexed Au-species and succeeded in finding a method of deactivation of the Hg-195m loaded column so that it could be eluted with THIO (10). A full description of these experiments is however beyond the scope of this chapter.

Column experiments with Hg-195m/Au-195m. The investigation was then directed primarily to the SiO_2-ZnS/THIO system, with the option that in the case of moderate or negative results, some other of the previously indicated systems would be tested. The experiments were carried out in three stages - preliminary and low activity experiments to establish a working technique and limiting conditions for the generator operation, scaling up for animal tests and, finally, construction of the hot-cell facilities and final design of the generator for human tests.

Production of Hg-195m. The Hg-195m parent isotope is prepared in the Philips Isochronous 30 MeV cyclotron in Petten by the Au-197 (p, 3n) Hg-195m + Hg-195 reaction. The irradiation with an internal 28 MeV proton beam is carried out on a 40-50 μm thick gold layer, electroplated on a copper support cooled with water. The proton energy is degraded in the gold layer to ca 17 MeV. Since gold is monoisotopic, under these conditions of irradiation no significant amounts of other mercury isotopes are produced, except for a small amount of Hg-197 which decays to stable Au-197. Typical production rates are 4.6 mCi Hg-195m and 12 mCi Hg-195 per μAh, respectively. The irradiated target is allowed to cool down for a variable time period, which ranged from 24-36 hours for the low activity experiments to several hours for the high activity experiments, to decrease the excess of Hg-195 ($T\frac{1}{2}$ 9.9.h). From the cooled target the gold layer is stripped mechanically and radioisotopes of mercury are separated from the Cu/Au chip by means of dry distillation. For the low activity experiments vacuum distillation with a liquid nitrogen cooled mercury collector (15) was used. Dry distillation working with carrier gas flow, sweeping the mercury vapours into a nitric acid scrubber, was used for high activity productions. The separation efficiency of the latter system is quantitative and the separation (including stripping) takes 15 minutes. The resulting solution of radioactive mercury in nitric acid is further formulated by diluting it with water for injections, followed by neutralization to almost neutral pH, to obtain the "loading solution" with the desired radioactive concentration.

Production of generator columns. The column body consists of 0.7 mm I.D. glass tube provided with a sintered glass filter and widened at each end to fit the standard 22 mm rubber stoppers. The columns are placed in the rack connected to a vibrator, filled partly with a neutral nitrate solution (of the same composition as loading solution) to which a thick slurry of the sorbent is added in portions under mild vibrations, until the settled bed reaches 2 mm from the upper widened portion. On the top of the sorbent bed is placed a porous polypropylene filter disc and a retaining ring. The head space is filled with nitrate solution, closed with a stopper and crimped. The columns are autoclaved and stored for use. A cross-section of the column is given in Figure 2.

For loading with radioactive mercury the colums were pre-washed with nitrate solution, loaded with 2-20 ml of the active solution and again washed with nitrate solution. Each fraction was allowed to pass through the column under gravity with flow rate 0.2-0.5 ml/min. Generators which were not sterilized were left in the loading rack and washed with eluent, generators which were sterilized, were removed from the rack and autoclaved in nitrate or other media.

Evaluation of the generator performance. Since the Hg/Au generator has been intended primarily for bolus operation (rapid single elution with a small volume of eluent) the elution system and the mode of operation were adjusted to this requirement. For the elutions the upper septum of each generator was connected via needles and thin silicone rubber tubing provided with a three-way membrane valve to the bottle with eluent. To the three-way valve was attached a 2 ml syringe, serving as a pumping device. The lower septum of each generator was connected via needles and tubing to a vial collecting the eluate. Each generator was eluted with 2.5 ml eluent (to correct for the dead volume of the outlet tubing) forced through the column in 3 - 4 seconds by means of the pumping syringe.

The collected eluate was placed in a standard geometry above the Ge-Li detector coupled to a fast single channel gamma analyzer controlled by two interconnected automatic timers - one setting the counting time (10 sec) and one controlling the repetition cycle (30 sec). Depending on the eluate activity, the first (10 sec) count started at an exact time after t_o (for instance 60 seconds) and was repeated in 30 sec intervals for 270 sec after t_o. The count rate of the 261 keV gamma ray was registered. In this way we determined the decay curve for each eluent. After correcting the registered count rates (for each interval) for the decay in the time elapsed from t_o and decay during the counting period (and other usual corrections) the mean of all values was taken as count rate at t_o and recalculated to the mCi of Au-195m per eluate at t_o. To compare directly the results of various elutions and the results obtained from various generators, corrected yields (mCi) were normalized to 14.00 h of the day of elution (corrected for $T\frac{1}{2}$ of Hg-195m). The relative percentage was calculated from the known Hg-195m activity loaded on the generators (1 mCi Hg-195m yields 0.458 mCi Au-195m) and the yield (mCi) of Au-195m. Each eluate was then counted (about 20 min. later) once more at 261 keV to determine the background originating from Hg-195m breakthrough (used as a correction for calculation of mCi Au-195m) and at 560 keV to determine the breakthrough of Hg-195m. This latter value was also normalized to 14.00 hours of the day of elution.

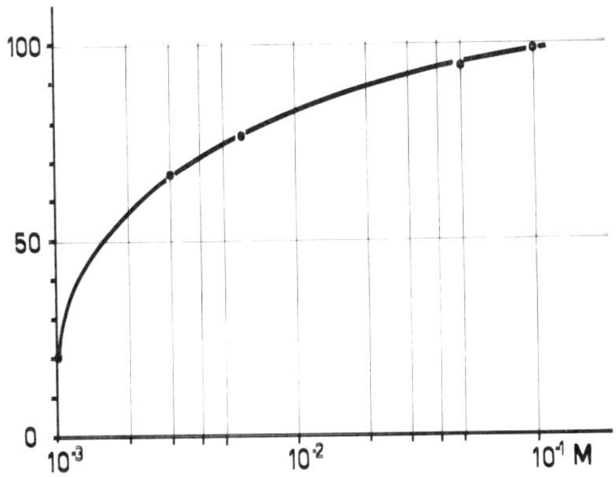

Figure 1. Simulated elution yield vs. molarity of the eluent. System SiO_2-ZnS/Au-198-THIO.

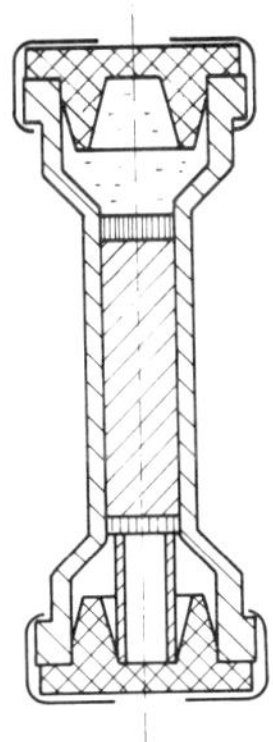

Figure 2. Cross section of the generator column.

Results and Discussion

The preliminary low activity experiments (1-15 mCi Hg-195m/generator) showed relatively low yields (10-40%) and poor reproducibility from generator to generator. Investigation of this phenomenon led to early discovery of two effects causing a distinct decrease in yield-sterilization by autoclaving, and a strong radiation effect. We found that the yield is inversely proportional to the total mercury activity absorbed on the generator as seen from Figure 3. The same Figure illustrates the negative effect of the excess of directly produced Hg-195 which strongly contributes to the absorbed radiation dose in generators produced shortly after EOB (lower line). In generators produced later after EOB, mostly close to the decay equilibrium of both mercury isotopes, the radiation contribution of Hg-195 is much lower (ca 0.7 mCi Hg-195/mCi Hg-195m), which results in an increased yield (upper line).

Eluent. When evaluating the various concentrations of THIO solutions as an eluent, we found that the yield of Au-195m depends on the THIO concentration similarly as shown in Figure 1. However, for the real parent/daughter pair, 97% "elution yield" is not reached, but, depending on the generator loading, only 25-45% (see Figure 3). An increase in THIO concentration to 0.2 M did not result in a better yield. Therefore, the concentration of THIO was adjusted to an isotonic concentration, 29.8 mg sodium thiosulphate pentahydrate per ml water for injection. It was also observed that generators allowed to stand in isotonic THIO overnight gave the following day lower yield than found earlier. The drop in yield was more pronounced for heavily loaded generators and reached only 70-40% of the first day values. Because it was thought impractical to change the generator medium for the night, we have tested a number of additives, known as effective scavengers, to counter the observed decrease. It was found that an addition of 1% sodium nitrate to the THIO solution stabilized the yield for four days. Sodium nitrite acted similarly giving the same to slightly higher (ca 3%) yields.

A separate problem is presented by the possible radiation decomposition of THIO. Thus it is reported that the main radiolytic products of THIO solution are sulphate, sulphur and sulphite with respective G values of 0.8; 0.55 and 0.16 and overall G decomposition value (-THIO) of 2.95 (16). A contradicting report (17) states that major radiolytic products are sulphur and hydrogen sulphide, which are however not observed when nitrite is added to the reaction system. The overall decomposition value G (-THIO) is in the latter case 0.7. Since nitrite and nitrate act in a similar way, the decrease in G (-THIO) can substantiate the addition of nitrate to our eluent, and possibly explain the stabilization of Au-195m elution yield as the result of lower G (-THIO). It has been of interest, however, to determine, what effect the radiolytic products could have on the performance of the generator, yield and Hg-breakthrough. Experiments with eluents to which a large excess (0.5% w/v) of respectively sulphate, sulphide and sulphite was added, showed that sulphate has little or no effect while sulphite and sulphide in large concentrations can cause a drastic decrease in yield (to 2-4% from 30-35% found in controls). Sulphide is especially harmful, causing also a considerable increase in Hg-breakthrough (0.16-0.25% vs. 0.005% in controls).

Since it was established that sodium thiosulphato aurate(I) complex is for all practical purposes not adsorbed on the SiO_2-ZnS sorbent, then the difference between the simulated and real generator yields indicates that in the real generator a competition probably exists between the sorbent and the eluent for the non-complexed Au-195m species. Although relatively little is known about the mechanism of thiosulphato aurate(I) complex formation, it has been suggested (18) that the reaction proceeds in several steps, with at least one step having a slower reaction rate. Because simple ionic forms of Au are strongly adsorbed on ZnS, it is possible that a fraction of some intermediate product (before being completely stabilized as thiosulphato aurate) is rapidly adsorbed on the sorbent and becomes nonelutable. In an attempt to affect the mechanism and the rate of thiosulphato aurate complex formation, a number of additions to the eluent were tested but without particular success. The investigation in this direction still continues.

Sorbent. In further sorbent experiments silica gel of various porosity, Controlled Pore Glass of various porosity, alumina and some special sorbents developed for HPLC (particularly pellicurar sorbents Chromosorb LC 2 and Perisorb A) were tested. All these carrier materials were coated with ZnS by means of the standard procedure described earlier (10). Standard SiO_2-ZnS sorbent, sieved to fractions with various particle sizes (0.075-0.200 mm) was also tested. The motivation behind all these experiments was the possible effect of the diffusion rate of Au-195m species and Au-195m thiosulphato aurate(I) complex on the supports. It was speculated that if the diffusion rate of the active species through the pores of the sorbent is, in comparison to the $T\frac{1}{2}$ of Au-195m, too slow, a fraction of Au-195m activity might decay before reaching the main body of the eluent. None of these experiments however produced any improvement in the elution yield. Similarly, variations in the concentration of ZnS (0.1-20 mg/g sorbent) did not produce any effect on the generator performance, except that losses of Hg-195m during loading of the generators were somewhat increased when working with sorbents low in ZnS content (0.1-0.5 mg/g).

Sterilization effect. Pharmaceutical requirements dictate that the generators be either aseptically produced or sterilized by autoclaving. This posed a problem because experiments with autoclaved generators showed decreased yields even for low active generators (30-25% vs. ca 40% for nonautoclaved controls). Because this effect was attributed to the thermal decomposition of THIO during autoclaving, experiments were carried out with sterilization of the generators in other media, namely chlorides, nitrates, sulphates, in various concentrations, including water for injections itself. We chose as the best compromise a solution of nitrate, having the same composition as the loading solution. However, to maintain the stability of elution yield, the generators sterilized in nitrate had to be aseptically washed with sterile eluent immediately after the autoclaving. The results obtained from generators produced in this way in comparison with nonautoclaved generators (dashed line) are illustrated in Figure 4. Most recently further improvement was achieved by sterilization of the generators in buffered THIO-nitrate eluent.

Design and performance of the generator for clinical tests. To make the generator for clinical tests safe for transportation and easy to use, a generator system was designed as illustrated in Figure 5. To make the assembly of the high activity generators easier the production procedure was slightly modified. The generator column loaded with Hg-195m was removed from the loading rack and inserted into a tightly fitting aluminium capsule provided with a fixed outlet elution needle protruding through the bottom of the capsule. On the top of the generator was placed a fitting aluminium cap provided with fixed inlet elution needle. Applying a mild pressure, the needles pierced the lower and upper septa of the generator column, closing it simultaneously tightly in the capsule. The capsule with the generator was then sterilized in the autoclave. Autoclaved capsules were placed in lead containers, each generator was aseptically washed with 15 ml of sterile eluent and sealed for transportation. Loading of the generators ranged from 380-470 mci Hg-195m (880-1100 mCi of both mercury isotopes) at the time of production at 14.00 hours on Monday. The generators were eluted with eluent as specified in Table VI. Control elutions were carried out with 2-2.5 ml at intervals of 3 to 5 minutes, a minimum of 20 times, and a maximum of 84 times per generator per day. The latter number of elutions corresponds approximately to the number of elutions needed for the clinical investigation of 6 patients per day, including the preelutions and control elutions between clinical applications.

In the collected eluates yields and Hg-195m-breakthroughs were determined as already described. The eluates were also analyzed for zinc content, pH, sterility and apyrogenicity. Typical properties of an eluate obtained from a 470 mCi generator are given in Table VII. The typical daily elution pattern - elutions of the same generator on Wednesday - is shown in Figure 6, mCi Au-195m per eluate (A) and Hg-195m breakthrough in μCi Hg-195m/mCi Au-195m (RN). From Figure 6 it is seen that the initial

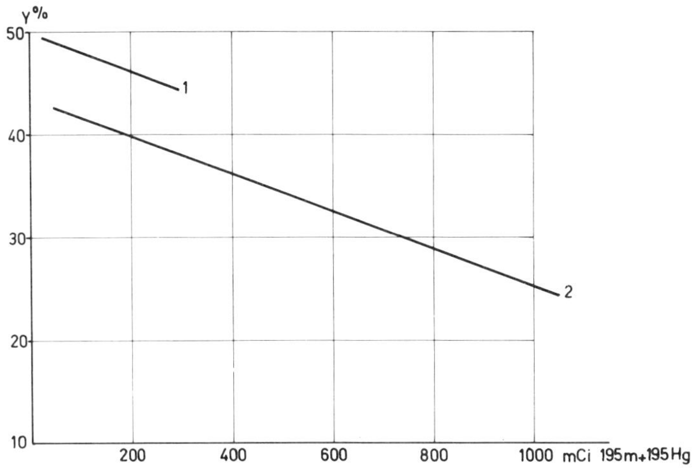

Figure 3. Elution yield of Au-195m vs. mercury activity (mCi) adsorbed on the column. Key: 1, generators produced 36 h or later after EOB; and 2, generators produced within 10 h after EOB.

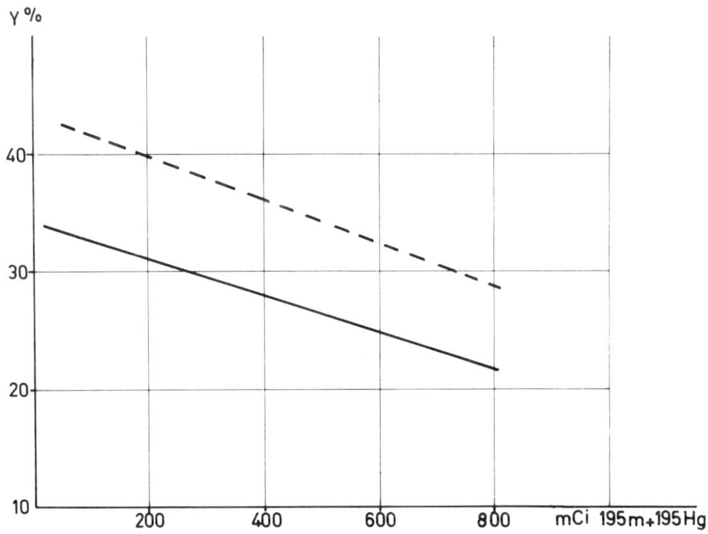

Figure 4. Elution yield of Au-195m. Generators autoclaved in nitrate solution. Dashed line: not autoclaved generators washed with THIO immediately after loading.

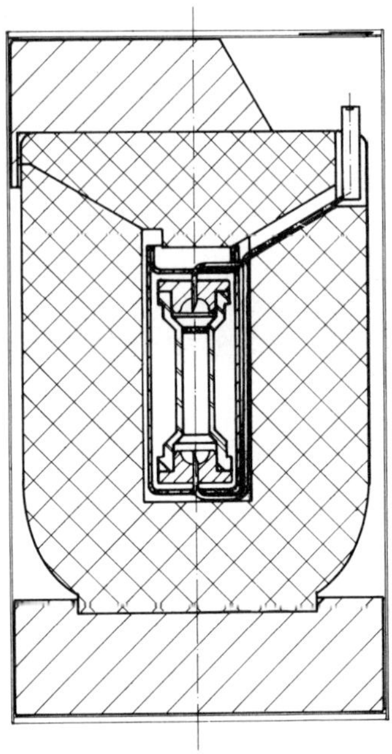

Figure 5. Cross section of the Hg-195m/Au-195m generator.

Table VI. Specifications of the Presently Used Eluent.

Composition	: 29.8 mg/ml sodium thiosulphate.5 H_2O 10.0 mg/ml sodium nitrate
pH	: 6 - 8
Osmotic Pressure	: 440-510 mOs (1.6 x isotonic)
Sterile	: complies with U.S.P.
Pyrogen free	: complies with U.S.P.

breakthrough is very rapidly washed off the column and is stabilized after about 15-18 elutions at 0.4-0.3 μCi Hg-195m/mCi Au-195m. The pattern of Hg-195m wash out (in % of the column loading) as shown in Figure 7, correlates well with the wash out of zinc (in μg Zn/ml eluate) which could possibly indicate radiation damage of ZnS (overnight) because the initial values of Zn concentration (first eluates) are much higher than the solubility of ZnS in a normal eluent (7.1 μg/ml) under the same circumstances. With this type of generators were carried out animal tests, pharmacology, toxicology, dosimetry and finaly successful human clinical tests, of which more detail description is however beyond the scope of this article.

Table VII. Properties of Eluate from 470 mCi Generator

Elution yields:		
1st day after production	40 ± 2 mCi Au-195m	(30 ± 1%)
2nd day after production	28 ± 1 mCi	(30 ± 1%)
3rd day after production	20 ± 1 mCi	(32 ± 2%)
4th day after production	14 ± 0.5 mCi	(33 ± 1%)
Radionuclidic purity	: Hg-195m <1 μCi/mCi Au-195m Au-195 <1.6 μCi total per 100 mCi Hg-195m present on the generator at time of elution	
pH	: 6 - 8	
Zinc content	: <5 μg/ml eluate	
Sterile	: complies with U.S.P.	
Pyrogen free	: complies with U.S.P.	

Summary

A Hg-195m/Au-195m generator has been developed for production of 30.6 second Au-195m radioisotope, useful for diagnostic application, particularly in cardiology. The generator is suitable for bolus injection and usable for at least three days, delivering sufficient activity of Au-195m (40-16 mCi per elution) in a

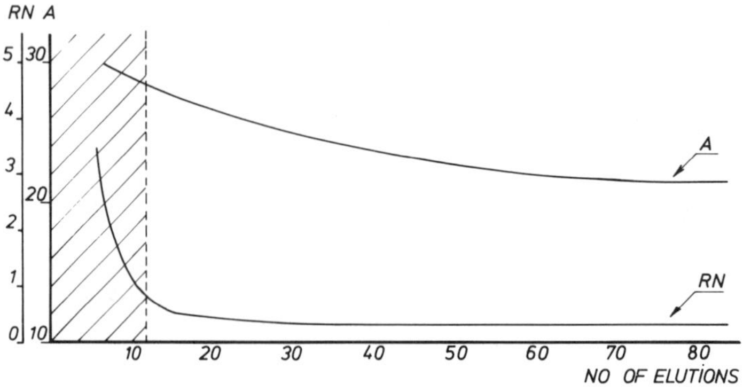

Figure 6. Elution pattern of 470 mCi generator. Key: A, mCi Au-195m per eluate; and RN, radionuclidic purity of eluates (μCi Hg-195m/mCi Au-195m).

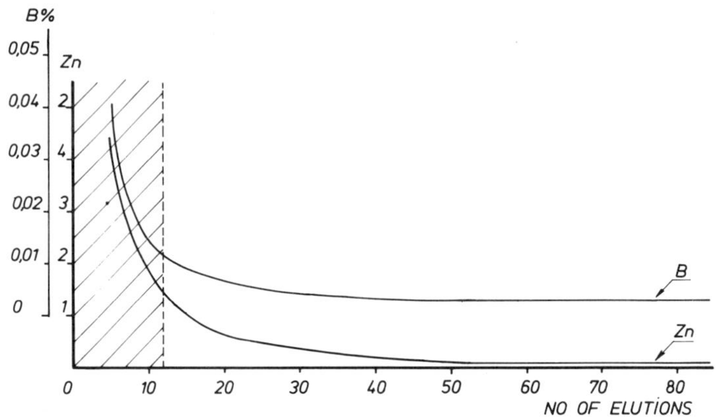

Figure 7. The pattern of Hg-195m breakthrough (B) in percent of Hg activity adsorbed on the column, and zinc washout (Zn) in μg/mL eluate.

nontoxic, pharmaceutically acceptable, sterile eluate. Clinical tests confirmed this generator as a valuable tool for dynamic studies.

Literature Cited

1. Campbell, E.C.; Nelson, F. J. Inorg. Nucl. Chem. 1956, 3, 233-242.
2. Yano, Y.; Anger, H.O. J. Nucl. Med. 1968, 9, 2-6.
3. Treves, S.; Kulprathipanja, S.; Hnatowich, D.J. Circulation 1976, 54, 275-279.
4. Jones, T.; Clark, J.C. J. Nucl. Med. 1970, 11, 118-124.
5. Madhusudhan, C.P. Proc. 173rd ACS Meeting 1977, Abstr. No.80.
6. Holman, B.L.; Harris, G.I.; Neirinckx, R.D.; Jones, A.G.; Idoine, J. J. Nucl. Med. 1978, 19, 510-513.
7. Lebowitz, E.; Richards, P. Seminars in Nucl. Med. 1974, 4, 257-268.
8. Yano, Y. in "Radiopharmaceuticals", Soc. Nucl. Med. Inc., New York 1975, 236-245.
9. Amphlett, C.B.; Mc Donald, L.A.; Redman, M.J. J. Inorg. Nucl. Chem. 1958, 6, 220-235.
10. Panek, K.J. Neth. Pat. Appl. No. 8002235, 16. April 1980
11. Leyden, D.E.; Luttrell, G.H.; Patterson, T.A. Analyt. Lett. 1975, 8, 51-56; Analyt. Abstr. 1975, 29, 3B7.
12. Coleman, G.H.; Bett, R.; Cuninghame, J.G.; Sims, H.E. Brit. Pat. Appl. P 8035352, 4 Nov. 1980.
13. Bett, R.; Coleman, G.H.; Cuninghame, J.G.; Sims, H.E. Nucl. Med. Comm. 1981, 2, 75-79.
14. Bett, R.; Cuninghame, J.G.; Sims, H.E.; Willis, H.H. Proc. 4th Int. Symp. on Radiopharmaceutical Chem. 1982, 173.
15. Wilkniss, P.E.; Beach, L.A.; Marlow, K.W. Radiochim. Acta 1972, 17, 110-113.
16. Natroshvilli, G.R.; Nanobashvilli, E.M. Chem. Abstr. 1970, 73, 40429 k.
17. Arnikar, H.J.; Patnaik, S.K.; Sarkhawas, D.B.; Pathak, T.P.S. Radiochim. Acta 1977, 24, 129-131.
18. Gjaldbaek, J.K. Dansk. Tids. Farm. 1927, 1, 251; Chem. Abstr. 1927, 21, 2443.

RECEIVED September 22, 1983

2

Usefulness and Performance of the Au-195m Generator

ISMAEL MENA and CAROL MARCUS—Department of Radiology, Division of Nuclear Medicine, Harbor-UCLA Medical Center, Torrance, CA 90509

ROLF DEJONG—Byk-Mallinckrodt, Petten, Holland

WALTER WOLF—Radiopharmacy Program, University of Southern California, School of Pharmacy, Los Angeles, CA 90033

Clinical usefulness of the Au-195m generator has been confirmed in several countries. The principal advantages are the reduction of patient radiation exposure and the possibilities of multiple, background-free, sequential evaluations of left and right ventricular function, both at rest and during exercise. Gold-195m has a half-life of 30.5 sec and is generator-produced from Hg-195m (T 1/2 = 41.6 hr). Mercury-195m is cyclotron-produced from an Au-197 target by the (p,3n) reaction during bombardment with 28.5 Mev protons. Mercury-195m decays by electron capture 45.8% of the time to Au-195m; 262 keV gammas are used for imaging. Breakthrough of the parent Hg-195m has two negative effects, since it increases patient exposure and degrades image quality due to high energy gammas. The breakthrough is 0.75 ± 0.09 μCi of Hg/mCi of Au-195m. The reproducibility of elution has a coefficient of variation of $2.5 \pm 0.3\%$. The eluates were sterile and pyrogen-free. The yield of the generator is 20-30 mCi of Au-195m from 155 mCi of Hg-195m generator. The short half-life of Au-195m offers the potential of frequent background-free determinations of left ventricular function which offer additional use for evaluation of left ventricular ejection fraction and volume indices. Rapid acquisition of data from varying levels of exercise, frequent assessment of pharmacologic and physiologic interventions and simultaneous acquisitions of data using more than one radionuclide become readily feasible with agents such as Au-195m.

0097-6156/84/0241-0023$06.00/0
© 1984 American Chemical Society

Ultra short-lived radionuclides are highly desirable for dynamic nuclear medicine studies. Such radionuclides offer multiple advantages, the most important of which are: a) bedside production from radionuclide generators; b) radiation exposure limited close to the time of measurement and therefore lowering markedly the exposure to the patient; c) administration of large mCi doses since high count rates can be detected by present-day digital and multicrystal cameras without significant coincidence losses; d) multiple, sequential background-free studies (e.g., Au-195m every 3 min); and e) the possibility of performing multiple radionuclide studies simultaneously. We have reported (1) the simultaneous use of Tl-201 and Au-195m for obtaining myocardial perfusion and ventriculographic information. After the simultaneous intravenous administration of both radionuclides, imaging of the right and left ventricles is performed for 30 sec using the Au-195m 260 keV spectrum without interference from the soft Tl-201 X-rays. After 5 min, Au-195m has decayed to undetectable levels, permitting routine Tl-201 imaging. We have also reported (2, 3, 4, 5) the rapid, sequential use of Au-195m and Tc-99m for both first-pass and ECG-gated equilibrium blood pool studies.

Among the clinically feasible ultra short-lived radionuclides, Au-195m offers distinct advantages for nuclear medicine, particularly in the area of nuclear cardiology. The Au-195m (T 1/2 = 30.5 sec) is available from a radionuclide generator (Figure 1). Its parent, Hg-195m (T 1/2 = 41.6 hr), is cyclotron-produced from an Au-197 target by the (p,3n) reaction during bombardment with 28.5 Mev protons (6). The Hg-195m decays by electron capture 45.8% of the time to Au-195m and by isomeric transition 54.2% of the time to Hg-195 (Figure 2). The useful energy of Au-195m is the 262 keV photon, produced in 68% of events. The fact that there is breakthrough of the parent Hg-195m in each elution makes it important to analyze the energies of radiation from Hg-195m, which decays 32.3% of the time by emission of a 262 keV gamma. There are higher gamma emissions also, at 388 keV (2.3%) and 560 keV (7.5%) (Table I). A high percentage of contamination with the parent Hg-195m would therefore significantly compromise image quality and increase radiation exposure dose to the patient. We wish to report on: 1) Measurements of Hg-195m breakthrough from Au-195m generators prepared by Byk-Mallinckrodt, Inc., 2) Reproducibility of elutions yield, and 3) Results of sterility and pyrogenicity studies performed in conjunction with human administration.

Experimental

Au-195m generator. The generator is currently available from Byk-Mallinckrodt, Inc. Petten, Holland, and from Mallinckrodt,

Inc., St. Louis, U.S.A. For details on yield, dimensions, absorbance, etc., please see the paper by Panek in this same volume.

Breakthrough of Hg-195m. The following technique was employed to measure Hg-195m breakthrough. Ten Au-195m generators were eluted consecutively with 2 ml of a solution containing sodium thiosulfate (29.8 g/l) and sodium nitrate 10 g/l). The elutions were performed every 3 min.; the initial three elutions were saved for counting in a NaI (Tl) well-type scintillation system. An additional 7 elutions were performed on each generator also every 3 min. Following this series, a 2 ml elution was diluted in 1,000 ml of water, and an aliquot of 1 ml. was placed in the well counter with the spectrometer set at 260 kev with a 10% window. Six-second counts were obtained every 30 sec for a period of 6 min, and, at the 7th min, a 1-min count was performed. Counts vs time were plotted on semilog paper and extrapolated to t = 0 (the time of elution). The counts at 7 min were assumed to be Hg-195m, since more than 10 half-lives of Au-195m had elapsed. These counts were expressed as a percentage of the counts at zero time. Using data (7) that Hg-195m has a 32.3% frequency of 262 keV gamma radiations and that Au-195m has a 68% frequency of 262 keV gamma radiations (per 100 disintegrations), the percentage counts of Hg-195m were multiplied by a factor of 68/32.3 = 2.1 in order to express the concentration of Hg-195m in each elution as μCi Hg-195m/mCi Au-195m. These measurements were performed daily during the first 3-4 days of generator life. Eluates from two generators were filtered through a Swinnex-25 or Melix GS 0.22 micron Millipore filter unit (Millipore Corp. Bedford, Mass.) flushed with 2 ml of water and diluted to 1,000 ml of water. One ml of this dilution was counted following the protocol outlined above.

Reproducibility of elution activity of Au-195m. A 2.5 x 1.3 cm heavily shielded NaI (Tl) detector with a 1 cm opening in the collimator was placed 20 cm from the outlet of the generator. This outlet was connected to the intravenous tubing inserted into an antecubital vein of the patient. The detector was connected to a spectrometer set at 260 keV with a 10% window. Three-second measurements were performed immediately after elution in groups of 6 elutions repeated every 3 min in each patient.

Sterility and pyrogenicity testing. For these tests, samples of eluates were obtained from 7 generators. Samples of the first elution and the final elution (48 hr after heavy clinical use) were obtained from two generators. All samples were submitted to a reference laboratory unaware of the sequence in which the samples were obtained. All elution samples were determined to be sterile and pyrogen-free.

Results

Breakthrough of Hg-195m. The average of 50 measurements revealed a Hg-195m breakthrough of 0.75 ± 0.09 μCi/mCi Au-195m. During the first day, the breakthrough was 1.13 ± 0.2 μCi; on the second day, 0.59 ± 0.02 μCi/mCi; on the third day, 0.88 ± 0.1 μCi/mCi; on the fourth day (2 generators), 1.16 ± 0.14 μCi/mCi (Figure 3). The diminution of radioactivity in these samples during the first 4 min after elution fit a single exponential function with a half-life of 30 sec (Figure 4). On the first day, the breakthrough levels were decreased to 0.53 ± 0.02 μCi by filtering the solution as described above. There was no significant effect of filtering on the second and third days, but on the fourth day, filtering decreased the breakthrough to 0.9 ± 0.08 μCi/mCi (Figure 3).

Breakthrough was very significant in the first, second and third eluates of the day. The first elution of day 1 was 39 ± 2.4 μCi/mCi; on day 2, 21.6 ± 4.7 μCi/mCi; on day 3, 19 ± 5.9 μCi/mCi (Figure 5). The breakthrough in the second elution of day 1 dropped to 17.4 ± 2 μCi/mCi; on day 2, 6.8 ± 1.4 μCi/mCi; on day 3, 4.77 ± 0.8 μCi/mCi. Breakthrough in the third elution of day 1 dropped very significantly to 6.5 ± 1.2 μCi/mCi; on day 2, 1.95 ± 0.3 μCi/mCi; on day 3, 1.58 ± 0.46 μCi/mCi. However, the breakthrough levels of the third elution were still significantly higher than those of later elutions obtained after 10 elutions, 3 min apart (Figure 3).

The patient radiation exposure from Au-195m is quite insignificant. According to Ackers et al. (7), 20 mCi of Au-195m delivers 0.78 mrad/mCi to the heart and 0.16 mrad/mCi to the kidneys. A significant dose is delivered to the kidneys by Hg-195m (including Hg-195), 12.4 mrads/ μCi. Assuming a conservative breakthrough of 1 μCi of Hg-195m/mCi Au-195m, a 20 mCi injection of Au-195m would result in 251 mrad to the kidneys, or 1.5 rad after 6 consecutive injections. In contrast, the radiation absorbed doses from a first-pass cardiac study using 15 mCi of Tc-99m sodium pertechnetate are 170 mrad whole body, approximately 1,900 mrad to thyroid and large intestine, 450 mrad to ovaries and 130 mrad to testes (8).

Reproducibility of elution activity of Au-195m. The reproducibility of the eluted Au-195m activity was evaluated from 81 sequential measurements obtained on-line from the intravenous tubing utilized for patient injections. The

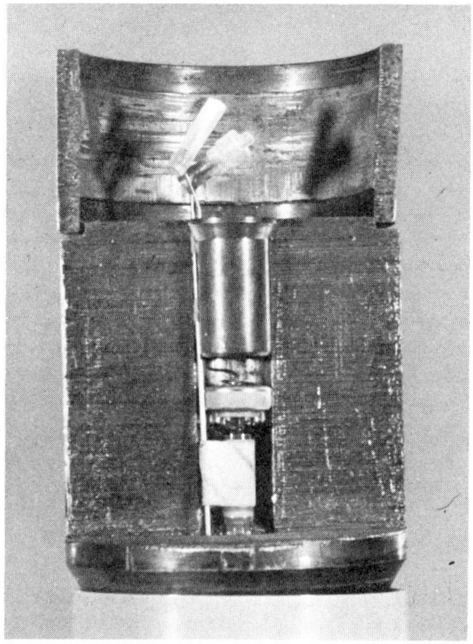

Figure 1. Hg-195m/Au-195m generator. ZnS-coated silica column heavily shielded in 360° . Circulation of eluate is from top to bottom.

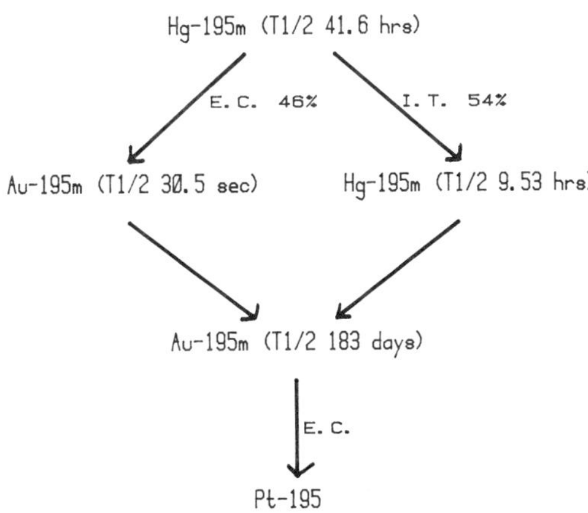

Figure 2. Decay scheme of Hg-195m. Notice decay to Au-195m and Hg-195, both radionuclides decay to Au-195.

Table I. Principal Gamma Emissions

	%	keV
Hg-195m	32.3	262
	2.3	388
	7.5	560
Au-195m	68	262

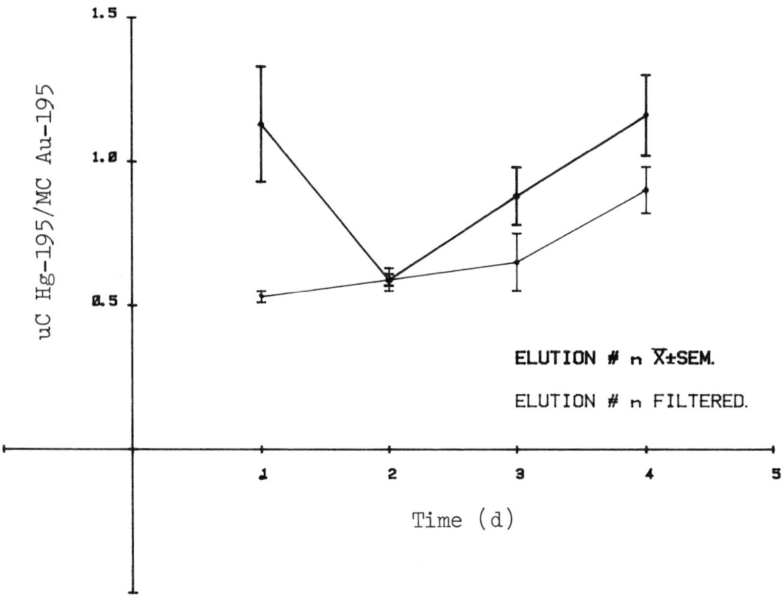

Figure 3. Breakthrough of Hg-195m. After 10 elutions, the breakthrough fluctuates between 1.1 μCi/mCi of Au-195m and 0.5 μCi/mCi of Au-195m. Significant effect is observed after Millipore filtration on day 1 and 4.

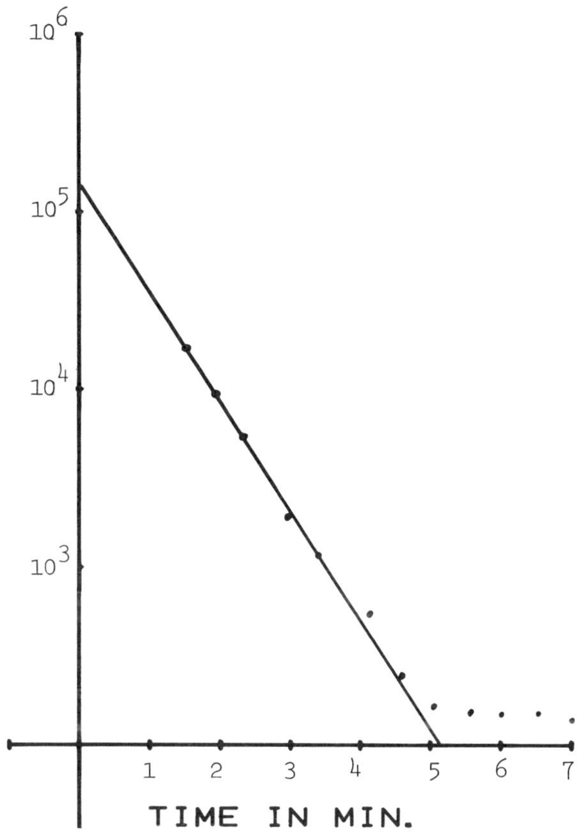

Figure 4. Exponential decay of eluate of Au-195m generator. T 1/2 is 30 sec, a residue of 0.03% of Hg-195m is detected at 5-7 min corresponding to Hg-195m/Au-195m breakthrough.

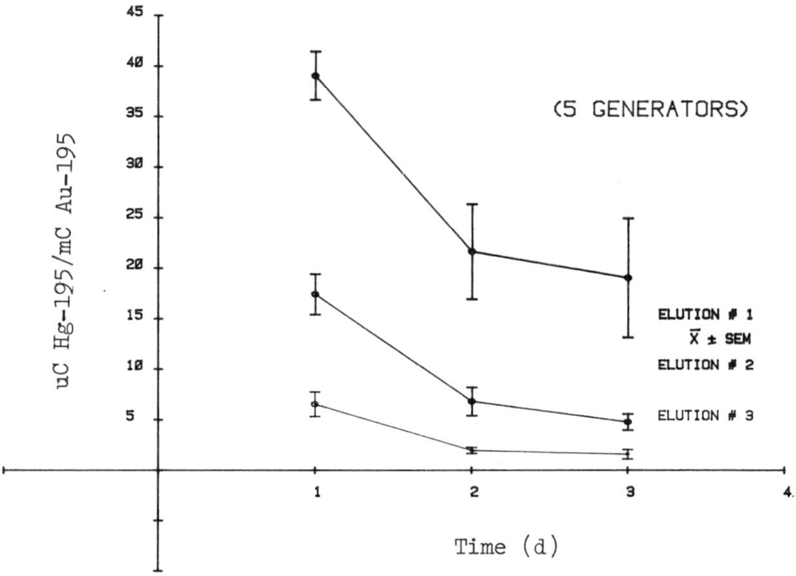

Figure 5. Breakthrough of Hg-195m in eluate of Au-195m generator. Notice large breakthrough in eluates 1 and 3 during the first 3 days of use of the generator.

coefficient of variation for the activity of Au-195m in the eluates was 2.5 ± 0.3%. While this degree of variation is quite acceptable, part of it may be due to the inherent variability of 3 cc disposable plastic syringes used routinely for clinical purposes.

Discussion

With presently available technology, the Au-195m generator demonstrates highly reproducible elution characteristics. Preliminary reports from other laboratories are consistent with our findings (9,10). The experimental evaluation and clinical use of the Au-195m generator presented here demonstrates the feasibility and potential usefulness of this short-lived radionuclide. The 30.5 sec half-life of this radionuclide has many obvious advantages. The generator reaches equilibrium rapidly after elution and may be eluted every 3-5 min at the bedside, as was accomplished in this study. The radiation exposure dose to the patient is substantially reduced with this agent as compared with Tc-99m, the conventional imaging agent. Based on the data presented in this evaluation, between 6 and 8 sequential Au-195m first-transit studies can be performed with radiation exposure closely equivalent to a single injection of 15 mCi of Tc-99m. The advantage of a 6-8 fold reduction in radiation exposure becomes even more important for applications in the pediatric age group, such as in pediatric cardiology. The radiation exposure from the Au-195m generator eluate is principally due to breakthrough of Hg-195m. Eluates for clinical purposes contained a mean of 0.7 μCi Hg-195m/mCi Au-195m.

As stated by the manufacturer, the first 10 elutions of the generator should be discarded. The first elution on day 1 particularly shows a very high level of Hg-195m breakthrough of 39 μCi/mCi, dropping to 20 μCi/mCi on days 2 and 3. The second and third elutions diminished rapidly to 15 and 16 μCi/mCi levels, respectively, and dropped further on days 2 and 3. However, these levels of mercury breakthrough are still unacceptable, and, for this reason, the manufacturer has recommmended discarding the first 10 elutions as a safety measure. This is a most important caveat which must be stressed to users of this generator.

The use of a 0.22 micron Millipore filter in preliminary studies resulted in lowered mercury breakthrough on day 1 of use and probably on day 4 as well. With the use of filters, breakthrough levels smaller than 0.6 μCi/mCi were obtained during the 3 days of generator use. These levels result in a significantly lower radiation exposure dose than has been calculated for an unfiltered breakthrough of 1 μCi/mCi. On day 4, the generator eluate is limited to non-cardiac studies because the activity of Au-195m is only about 6-8 mCi. This is sufficient, for example, for radionuclide venography.

The absolute yield of the generator has been estimated to be between 20-30 mCi of Au-195m with a 2 ml elution from a 155 mCi generator. At present, a convenient method for measuring the activity of Au-195m actually eluted from the generator at the beside is not available. We had made estimates using our Rad-X ionization chamber and a Selenium-75 standard. We observed very good reproducibility from multiple measurements of the same generator. These data were reported by the manufacturer during the pre-clinical trial period and were confirmed by the performance of generators retained by the manufacturer from the batches used in this study. Two generators out of a batch-size of 5 were retained by the manufacturer for analysis. They were eluted in a manner at times similar to those of our clinically used generators. The yields of Au-195m were measured with a Ge (Li) spectrometer with a known calibration factor at 262 keV, and the activities were extrapolated to time = 0 (beginning of elution).

The stability and reproducibility of the generator has been highly satisfactory. We have been able to sequentially study right and left ventricular function and segmental wall motion at different levels of exercise-induced stress. These results have been compared with simultaneously gathered data on myocardial perfusion with Thallium-201. This combination is made possible by the use of the short-lived Au-195m and provides studies of high sensitivity and specificity for the diagnosis and evaluation of patients with coronary artery disease. The sterility and pyrogenicity test results were satisfactory, and no untoward reactions have been noted during clinical use of this generator.

The availability of frequent background-free determinations of left ventricular function will open additional uses for evaluation of the left ventricular ejection fraction and volume indices. Rapid data acquisition at varying levels of exercise, frequent assessment of pharmacologic and physiologic interventions, and simultaneous acquisition of data using more than one radionuclide becomes readily feasible with agents such as Au-195m.

Acknowledgments

The authors wish to acknowledge the expert technical support of Mr. Jim Fain, R.T., Mr. Sammy Losiri, R.T., and the computer programming expertise of Mr. Craig Thompson.

Literature Cited

1. Mena, I.; Narahara, K.A.; Brizendine, M.;Carmody, J.; Maublant, J. Circulation 1982, 66, II-273.
2. Mena, I.; Narahara, K.A.; deJong, R.; Maublant, J. J. Nucl. Med. 1983, 24, 139-144.
3. Jengo, J.A.; Mena, I.; Blaufuss, A.; Criley, J. M. Circulation 1978, 57, 326-332.
4. Garcia, E.; Mena, I.; deJong, R.; Fain, J. J. Nucl. Med. 1981, 22, 71.
5. Mena, I.; deJong, R.; Mena, F.J.; Narahara, K.A. Proceedings of the International Symposium on Short-lived Radionuclides, Department of Energy, Washington, D.C., May 1982, in press.
6. Panek, K.J.; Lindeyer, J.; vander Vlugt, H.C. J. Nucl. Med. 1982, 23, 108.
7. Ackers, J.G.; deJong, R. J. Nucl. Med. 1982, 23, 68.
8. MIRD/dose estimate report #8. Summary of current radiation dose estimates to normal humans from 99mTc as sodium pertechnetate. J. Nucl. Med. 1976, 17, 74-77.
9. Wackers, F.; Giles, R.; Hoffer, P.; Lange, R.; Berger, H.; Zaret, B. J. Nucl. Med. 1982, 23, 48.
10. Wackers, F.J.; Giles, R.W.; Hoffer, P.B.; Lange, R.C.; Berger. H.J.; Zaret, B.L. Am. J. Cardiol. 1982, 50, 89-94.

RECEIVED September 22, 1983

3

Preparation and Characteristics of a Hg-195m/Au-195m Generator for First-Pass Angiography

R. BETT, J. G. CUNINGHAME, H. E. SIMS, and H. H. WILLIS—Atomic Energy Research Establishment, Harwell, Oxfordshire, OX11 0RA, England

D. S. DYMOND, W. FLATMAN, and D. L. STONE—St. Bartholomew's Hospital, West Smithfield, London EC1A 7BE, England

A. T. ELLIOTT—Western Infirmary, Glasgow, G11 6NT, Scotland

A Hg-195m/Au-195m generator has been developed for medical use in first pass heart angiography. The mercury parent is bound to a thiol-containing column material from which Au-195m is eluted in dilute sodium cyanide solution. Such generators may have large quantities of activity adsorbed on the column and this can result in radiolytic reactions which cause a decrease of elution efficiency with time. Careful timing of the various operations involved in preparing these generators can help to stop this deterioration. Gold-195m decays to Au-195 which has a half-life of 183 days and it is important to operate the generator in such way as to keep the amount of Au-195 injected into the patient to a minimum. The method of production of these generators is presented. Effects of radiolytic reactions on generator use, and implications of the mass 195 decay chain to ultimate purity of the product are discussed.

First pass radionuclide angiography of the heart involves the injection of a small bolus of radioactivity into a peripheral vein, and imaging the bolus as it passes through the heart. In recent years the quantitative measurement of cardiac function with this technique has become clinically useful in the assessment of cardiac disease (1). A major strength of the method is the ability to study cardiac physiology non-invasively under stress such as exercise, an approach which is diagnostically useful particularly in patients with coronary artery disease. A major drawback with the method is the requirement of a separate injection of the radionuclide for each study. Until recently the only available isotope for such studies has been Tc-99m, but its relatively long half-life (6 hours), along with the amount of activity required for each study (>10mCi), has precluded more than two injections per session because of patient dose and degradation of pictures by background activity in the blood pool. These restrictions have

0097-6156/84/0241-0035$06.00/0
Published 1984 American Chemical Society

prevented similar studies being carried out on paediatric patients where they could be used to identify valve disorders etc., since they would receive too high a dose. For the full potential of the technique to be realized a short lived isotope was required which would by necessity be the daughter of a long-lived parent, together making a generator pair.

Two such generator pairs have been previously reported: Rb-81/Kr-81m (2) and Os-191/Ir-191m (3), however neither is suitable since Kr-81m is eliminated from blood on passage through the lungs, and the half-life of Ir-191m (5 secs) is too short to permit adequate study of the left heart. However Lebowitz (4) noted the possibilities of the Hg-195m/Au-195m pair and we have already described our preliminary results (5,6) using this system. Another Hg-195m/Au-195m generator is also in clinical use (7). One based on a Chelex-100 resin has been reported (8), but no indication of activity on the column nor in solution was given. The characteristics for an ideal generator pair for first pass angiography and those of the Hg-195m/Au-195m generator described here are shown in Table I. The energy of the principal γ-ray

Table I. Physical Requirements of a Generator Pair for First Pass Angiography

Property	Ideal Generator	Hg-195m/Au-195m
Parent half-life	> 24 h	41 h
Daughter half-life	< 1 min	30.5 sec
Principal γ-ray	100-300 keV	262 keV
Abundance	100%	67%

(262 keV) is a little high and the abundance lower than ideal, but this system is nevertheless quite adequate. Operating requirements of a generator for the first pass angiography are shown in Table II. In practice the generator is likely to be based on a chromatographic column because of the short time available for anything other than a straight elution stage. The remainder of this paper describes the preparation and properties of such a generator with special reference to breakthrough and ultimate daughter impurities.

Experimental

Production of Hg-195m. Gold is monoisotopic and the most convenient method for preparation of Hg-195m is by the Au-197(p,3n) Hg-195m reaction. We irradiate metallic gold targets 0.5mm thick with 34 MeV protons. About 8 MeV is absorbed in the target, giving a practical yield of about 4 mCi/μA/hr at end of bombardment. Good cooling is essential to prevent loss of product during the irradiation because of the volatility of mercury. Mercury-195m is then separated from the gold target by placing in a furnace at 1000°C in a helium gas flow (50 ml/min) for 1 hour. The evaporated mercury is collected in 20 ml of nitric acid (10%) and then buffered with sodium acetate (5 g).

Table II. Operating Requirements of a Generator for First Pass Angiography

a)	Fast daughter/parent separation
b)	Daughter obtainable in good yield
c)	Daughter activity 10-20 mCi in 0.5 ml
d)	Low parent breakthrough
e)	Stable against radiation damage
f)	Daughter activity in non-toxic, pyrogen-free, sterile solution
g)	Robust for transport
h)	Easy to use

Column Adsorption of Hg-195m. Preliminary work and a review of the literature showed that conventional ion exchangers would not effect the separation of mercury and gold and that the best method would be to use an ion exchange material where the active species was a thiol group (9). The first material used was vicinal dithiocellulose (10), which has been described previously (5). This material had several disadvantages: it is not commercially available, it has high susceptibility to radiation damage and poor flow characteristics. Two additional commercially available thiol-containing materials were investigated and subsequently used in patient trials: they were thiopropyl sepharose-6B (Pharmacia Chemicals, Ltd.) and controlled pore glass (CPG) lipoamide (Pierce Chemical Co. Ltd.). These materials were prepared for use by washing with ethylene-diamine-tetraacetic acid/sodium acetate solution to chelate any heavy ions. This treatment also serves as a swelling solution for the sepharose material. The material was then reduced with mercapto-acetic acid for about 1 hour to produce free thiol groups and then washed several times with acetic acid/sodium chloride solution. Mercury-195m was then bound to the column material by mixing with the active solution and stirring by bubbling a slow gas flow through the solution for about 30 minutes. Mechanical stirring was found to increase parent breakthrough probably as a result of mechanical damage to the material resulting in small fragments passing through into the eluate. The material was then drawn onto the column and washed with about 50 ml of sodium cyanide (2.5 mM). Another material, Enzacryl polythiol (Koch Light Ltd.), was also investigated. This is a polymeric material which binds Hg very well, but undergoes radiolytic reactions turning it into a gel, which completely stops the passage of eluant through the material. It was found that drawing the active solution through the column material was also an excellent way of binding the mercury, except that it adsorbed in a very narrow band of extremely high "specific activity" ("specific activity" is used here as a measure of activity per mg of column material) which resulted in radiolytic reactions, causing a dramatic drop in elution efficiency.

Discussion

Column Performance. The only eluant found to elute Au-195m in any reasonable yield was NaCN, consequently the materials were investigated for variation in elution efficiency as a function of several variables, namely, concentration of cyanide, the volume of cyanide, and time/"specific activity" of Hg-195m on column. These parameters were of particular importance because of the over-riding requirement that the specific activity of Au-195m in solution should be greater than 20 mCi/ml. The parameter used to compare results was the % elution efficiency where:

$$\%\ \text{elution efficiency} = \frac{\text{Au-195m eluted} \times 10^2}{\text{Au-195m on column}}$$

The effect of cyanide concentration is shown in Figure 1. In order to keep the concentration of cyanide as low as possible, 2.5 mM was chosen for subsequent tests. Obviously higher efficiencies could be obtained with 10 mM cyanide - this would still be non-toxic under the clinical conditions used. Figure 2 shows the effect of varying cyanide volume on elution efficiency; clearly the smaller the volume of eluant the lower the elution efficiency. Conversely, the smaller the column the greater the efficiency, but all columns were >20% efficient with 0.6 ml of eluant. The volume of column material is controlled by the third parameter, that is the variation in elution efficiency with time for various "specific activities" of Hg-195m. Ideally there should be no variation in elution efficiency with time. The effect of varying "specific activity" is shown in Figures 3 and 4. These graphs show that at high "specific activities", although the initial elution efficiency may be very high it then drops, especially on standing overnight. This drop in elution efficiency was shown to be a result of radiolytic reactions by irradiating low "specific activity" columns in a Co-60 source. The results are shown in Table III. This mechanism is further confirmed by the suppression of damage by the use of radical scavengers. Table IV shows the radical and molecular products of water radiolysis along with their relative yields for gamma rays (11).

Some possible reactions which may be occurring are considered later in this paper. Any radionuclidic impurity will also contribute to this damage and since Hg-195 is produced directly during the irradiation as well as from the decay of Hg-195m (Figure 5), it is worth leaving the irradiated target for 10 to 20 hours before processing and loading the column.

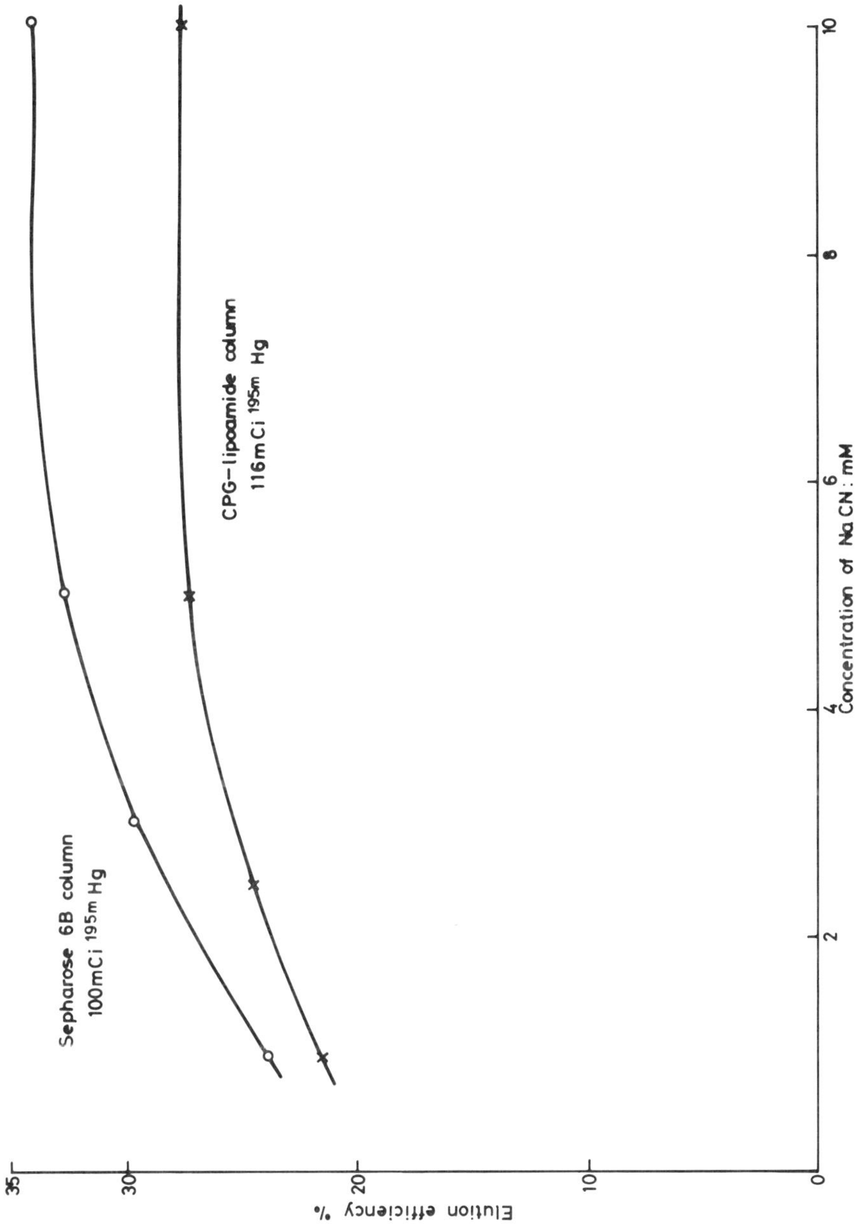

Figure 1. Variation of elution efficiency with concentration of cyanide.

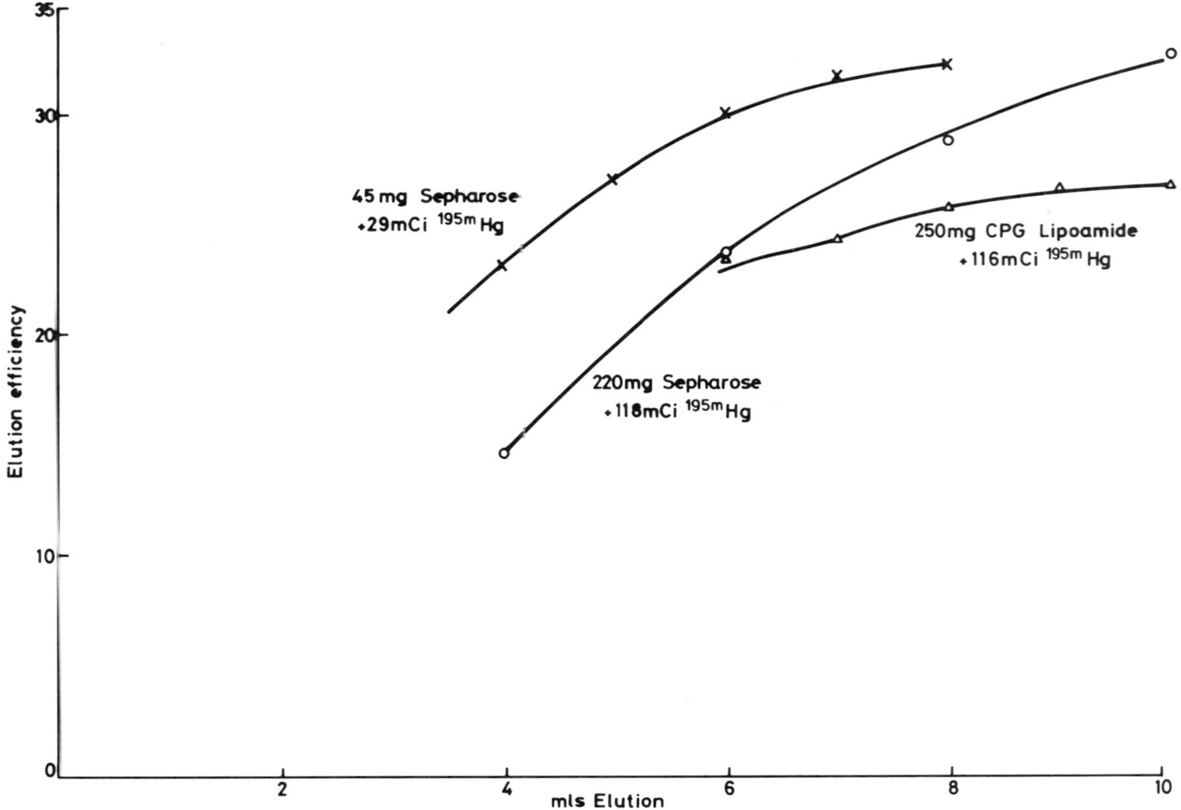

Figure 2. Variation of elution efficiency with volume of cyanide for Sepharose and CPG columns.

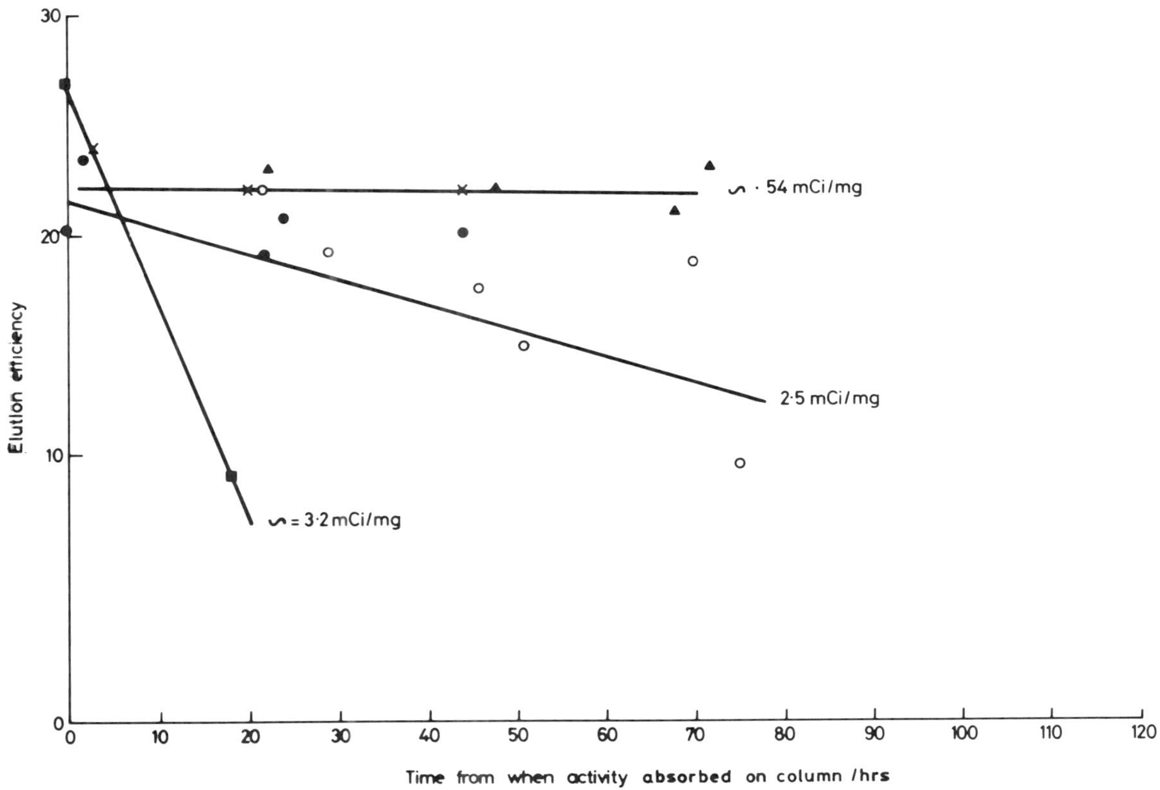

Figure 3. Sepharose Columns: Time dependence of elution efficiency for different "specific activity" columns.

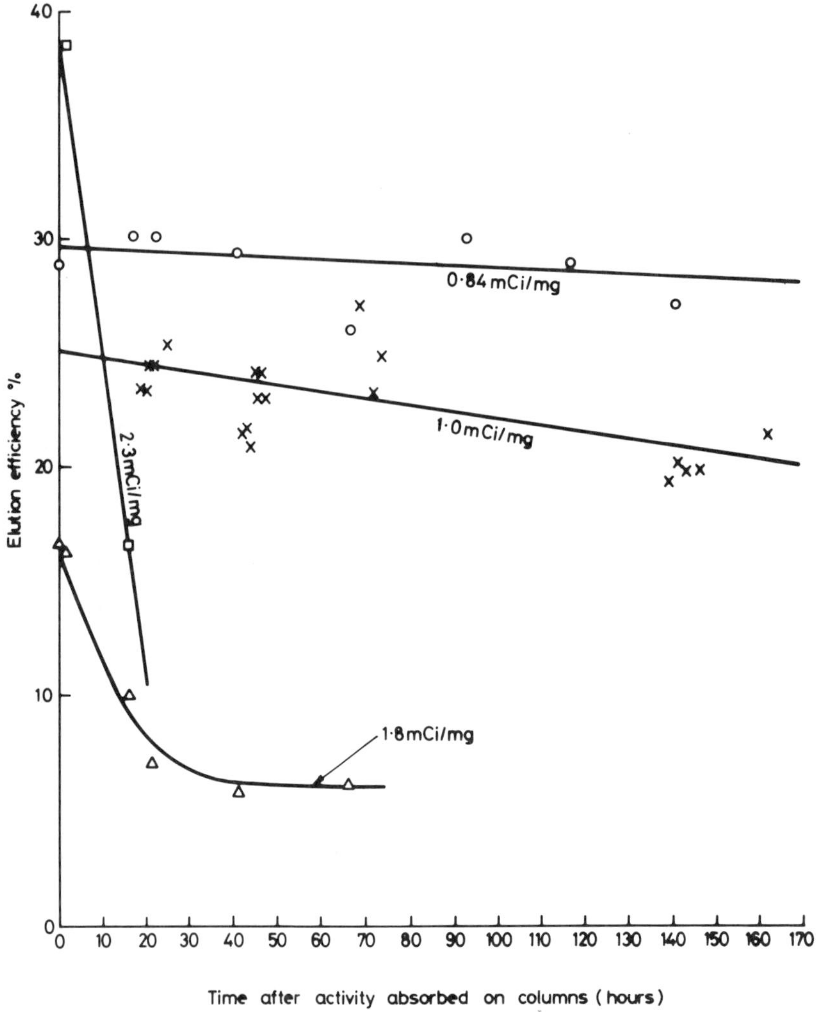

Figure 4. CPG Lipoamide Columns: Time dependence of elution efficiency for different "specific activity" columns.

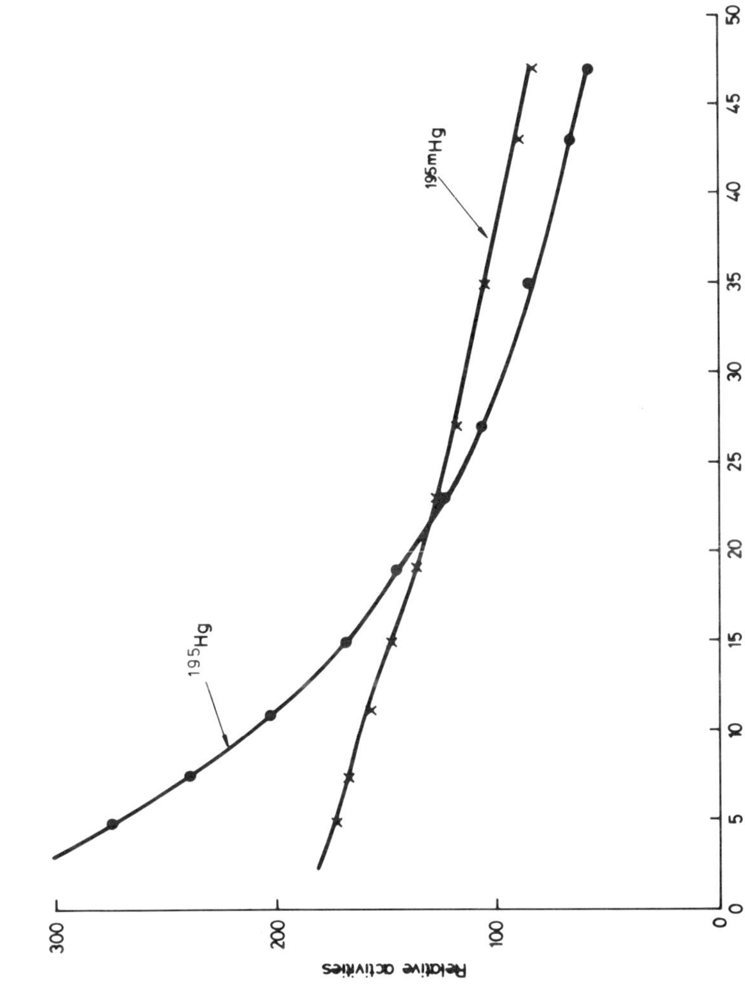

Figure 5. Variation of activity of Hg-195 and Hg-195m with time after EOB.

Table III. Effect of γ-Irradiation on Elution Efficiency

Experiment 1: Column Irradiated for Different Times

Dose (M Rad)	Elution Efficiency %	Hg-195m Breakthrough (μCi per mCi Au-195m)
0	56	3.0
0.16	56	2.4
3.2	35	0.8
13.4	11	0.8

Experiment 2: Comparison of Two Identical Columns

Dose	Efficiency	Breakthrough	Dose	Efficiency	Breakthrough
0	81	0.5	0	98	0.18
0	92	0.9	3.2	33	2.1
0	94	0.4	3.2	33	1.3*
0	80	0.2	3.2	14	0.8**
3.2	37	0.12	0	14	0.5

* Both columns eluted with 2% nitrate/2.5 mM cyanide
** Both columns eluted with 2.5 mM cyanide

Table IV: Radical and Molecular Products of Water Radiolysis

Species	No. formed per 100 eV absorbed
OH•	2.9
e^-	2.7
H•	0.6
H_2O_2	0.8
H_2	0.45

Breakthrough and Daughter Activities. The ideal column would have no breakthrough and the daughter would decay to a stable product. These generators do have a little breakthrough and Au-195m decays to Au-195 (see Figure 6) with a half-life of 183 days. On standing for any significant length of time (>20 mins) both sepharose and CPC lipoamide columns have a similar tendency: that is, the amount of Hg-195m in solution builds up as shown in Table V. Conversely, this level decreases to very low values with repeated use. Another point worth noting is the build up of the radioactive Au-195 with

Table V: Variation of Hg-195m Breakthrough with Time

Type of Column	Time Since Last Elution	Breakthrough μCi Hg-195m/mCi Au-195m
Sepharose (successive elutions)	5 min	0.75
	3 min	0.32
	3 min	0.21
	3 min	0.2
	3 min	<0.1
	3 min	
	3 min	
Lipoamide (successive elutions)	24 hr	50
	10 min	1
	10 min	<0.5

time. Whereas 1 mCi of Au-195m eluted from the column produces about 2 nCi of Au-195, it can be calculated that a column containing 100 mCi of Hg-195m will produce about 600 nCi Au-195 in 2.5 minutes (which is the average time between patient injections). In the course of 6 injections about 3-4 μCi Au-195 will thus be injected into patients. This will concentrate in liver and kidneys (about 80%) and bone and soft tissue (about 20%) (12). Any greater delay will result in a proportional build up of activities, so the columns should be eluted several times following a period when not in use. Furthermore, to keep the radionuclidic purity high the columns should be eluted again immediately after the sample for injection. Table V emphasizes this need for a strict protocol when operating these generators. If left standing for 30 minutes a 20 mCi generator produces 2 μCi Au-195 whereas washing at 10 minute intervals reduces the Au-195 level to 500 nCi. The high activity column shows results close to those calculated.

Chemical Aspects of the Columns. So far no mention has been made of the chemistry of the separation process on the column, nor of the nature of the radiolytic reactions inhibiting the elution. Some of the possible reactions are shown in Figure 7. It is assumed that mercury binds to the thiol as a "half salt" (reaction 1). The column then takes about an hour to reach its maximum elution efficiency. We assume that reaction 2 is taking place in this time and that this is a slow reaction. When Hg-195m decays by electron capture this will probably be accompanied by emission of one or more Auger electrons so the gold initially in the unstable +2 oxidation state will become +3. The elution step is probably the result of the stability constant of the cyanide complex being greater than the sulphur complex. There is also the possibility that a high charge as a result of the Auger process causes the Au-S bond to rupture after charge redistribution. Both these mechanisms

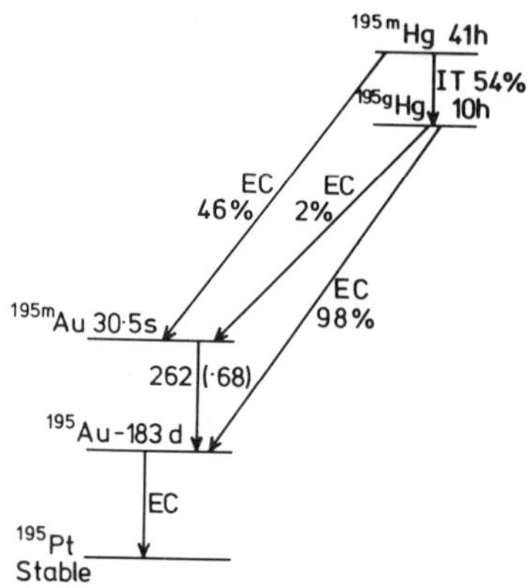

Figure 6. Hg-195m simplified decay scheme

Binding Stage

$$Hg(OAC)_2 + R\text{-}S\text{-}H \longrightarrow R\text{-}S\text{-}Hg\,OAC \quad R = \begin{cases} CPG \\ Sepharose \end{cases} \qquad 1$$

$$R\text{-}S\text{-}Hg\,OAC + CN^- \longrightarrow R\text{-}S\text{-}HgCN + {}^-OAC \qquad 2$$

Elution Stage

$$R\text{-}S\text{-}Hg\text{-}CN \longrightarrow R\text{-}S\text{-}Au\text{-}CN \qquad 3$$

$$\text{or} \longrightarrow R\text{-}S\text{-}Au^+\text{-}CN + \text{Auger Electron}$$

$$R\text{-}S\text{-}Au^+\text{-}CN \longrightarrow (Au(CN)_4)^{n-} \qquad 4$$

Possible Radiolytic Reactions

$$R\text{-}S\text{-}Hg\text{-}CN + e^- \longrightarrow R\text{-}S\text{-}Hg + CN^- \qquad 5$$

$$O_2 + e^- \longrightarrow O_2^- \qquad 6$$

$$R\text{-}S\text{-}Hg\text{-}CN + O_2^- \longrightarrow R\text{-}S\text{-}Hg + CN^- + O_2 \qquad 7$$

Figure 7. Some chemical reactions occurring on the columns.

are speculative. The nature of the radiolytic reactions are even more speculative, but one possibility is that the mercury in the +2 oxidation state is reduced to +1 by reactions such as 5-7 (Figure 7) and that the resulting gold-sulphur complex is stronger than the corresponding +2 or +3 complexes mentioned above. Although the column is only 25% efficient in eluting Au-195m it is 100% efficient in eluting Au-195.

Mechanical Aspects of Generator Design. In Table II the requirements of a generator are listed including the optimal volume of eluant should be about 0.5 ml, and that the generator should also be robust for transport and easy to use. The first requirement means essentially no dead volume in the system. Original designs were based on a modified isotope vial with a Luer fitting into an automatic valve into which a syringe could be inserted to draw off the activity for injection. This design, shown in Figure 8, is now being modified to make it more robust, although this system has stood up to road, rail and air transport without any problems.

Clinical Operation and Applications. A large number of tests on these generators has now been performed on both animals and humans. The generators are sterile, non-pyrogenic and very importantly, non toxic. Measurements have shown that administration of the cyanide containing eluate has not caused a measurable increase in plasma cyanide, red cell cyanide, or plasma thiocyanate levels, even when large volumes are administered (13,14). The levels remain within the normal range for non-smoking humans. In practice a catheter is inserted into a patient's forearm and connected to a short length of tube (vol. about 0.6 ml) with Luer fittings at both ends and terminating in a 3 way valve, one side of which is connected to a syringe containing 20 ml of saline. The remaining arm of the valve is used to inject the activity so as to just fill the tube. This is followed by the 20 ml of saline to force the bolus of activity into the vein. After investigating various automatic methods this proved still to be the simplest and safest method. Measurements of cardiac function have agreed closely with those obtained using Tc—99m (13,14) and Au-195m is now being used for rapid sequential radionuclide first pass angiography to assess evolutionary changes in cardiac function occurring after pharmocological or physiological interventions. The multiple data points that may be obtained with Au-195m were previously not possible with the first pass technique.

Summary

A generator has been produced which is capable of producing 10-20 mCi of Au-195m in about .6 ml. If care is taken in column use there is less than .2 μCi Hg-195m/mCi Au-195m in the eluant. The generator has proved robust for transport and easy to use, and reliable, allowing tests involving over 200 patients.

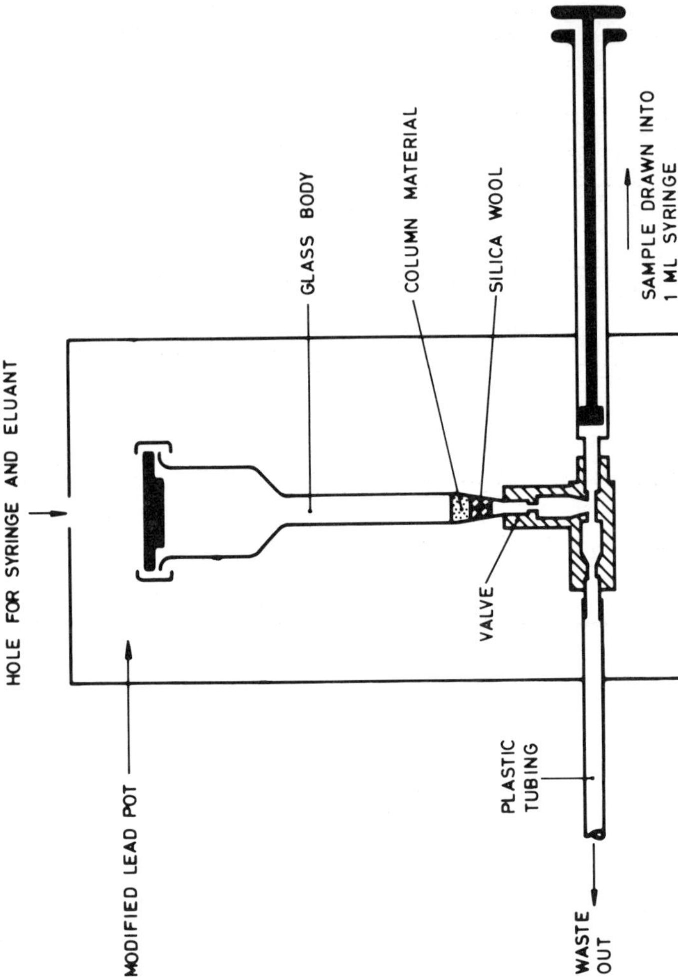

Figure 8. Schematic diagram of Hg-195m/Au-195m generator.

Acknowledgments

We gratefully acknowledge the help of Professor G. H. Coleman in the early stages of this work, and also D. L. Stone, P. L. Evans and D. Cooper - students who have all contributed greatly to this work. Finally our thanks are due to the Variable Energy Cyclotron staff for providing proton beams on demand and for manufacture of targets and other apparatus.

Literature Cited

1. Dymond, D.S.; Jarrett, P.H.; Britton, K.E.; Spurrell, R.A.J. Br. Heart Journal 1979, 41, 68-78.
2. Jones, T.; Clarke, J.C. Br. J. Radiol. 1969, 42,237.
3. Cheng, C.; Treves, S.; Samuel, A.; Davis, M.A. J. Nucl. Med. 1980, 21,1169-1176.
4. Lebowitz, E.; Richards, P. Semin. Nucl. Med. 1974, 4,257-268.
5. Bett, R.; Coleman, G.H.; Cuninghame, J.G.; Sims, H.E; Elliott, A.T.; Stone, D.L. Nucl. Med. Commun. 1981, 2,75-79.
6. Bett, R.; Cuninghame, J.G.; Sims, H.E.; Willis, H.H.; Dymond, D.S.; Flatman, W.; Stone, D.L.; Elliott, A.T. Int. J. Appl. Radiat. Isot. 1983, 34,959-963.
7. Panek, K.J.; Lindyer, J.; Van Der Vlugt, H.C. This volume.
8. Brihaye, C.; Guillaume, M.; Lavi, N.; Cogneau, M. J. Nucl. Med. 1982, 23,1114-1120.
9. The Radiochemistry of Mercury NAS-NS-3026.
10. Marchant, W. Environ. Sci. and Tech. 1971, 8,993-996.
11. Spinks, J.W.T.; Woods, R.J. "An Introduction to Radiation Chemistry"; 2nd edition; Wiley-Interscience, New York, 1976.
12. Newton, D.; Sims, H.E. Measurements being carried out at A.E.R.E. Harwell.
13. Elliott, A.T.; Dymond, D.S.; Stone, D.L.; Flatman, W.; Bett, R.; Cuninghame, J.G.; Sims, H.E.; Willis, H.H. Phys. Med. Biol. 1983, 28,139-147.
14. Dymond, D.S.; Elliott, A.T.; Flatman, W.; Stone, D.; Bett, R.; Cuninghame, J.G.; Sims, H.E. J. Amer. College of Cardiol., in press.

RECEIVED October 17, 1983

4

Chemical and Physical Parameters Affecting the Performance of the Os-191/Ir-191m Generator

A. B. PACKARD, S. TREVES, and G. M. O'BRIEN
Children's Hospital/Harvard Medical School, Boston, MA 02115

F. F. KNAPP, JR. and T. A. BUTLER
Oak Ridge National Laboratory, Oak Ridge, TN 37830

The development of an Os-191/Ir-191m generator suitable for radionuclide angiography in humans has elicited much interest. This generator employs "$[OsO_2Cl_4]^{2-}$" on AG MP-1 anion exchange resin with a Dowex-2 scavenger column and is eluted with normal saline at pH 1. The parent Os species is, however, neither well-defined nor homogeneous leading to less than optimal breakthrough of Os-191 (5×10^{-3}%) and modest Ir-191m yield (10-15%). The effect of a range of parameters on generator performance has been evaluated as has been the way in which the assembly and loading process affects generator performance. In addition, a number of potential alternative generator systems have been evaluated.

Ultra short-lived radionuclides offer a number of advantages over longer lived isotopes (such as Tc-99m) for angiocardiography. Some of these advantages include the ability to obtain serial images without increased background, higher photon flux, and lower patient radiation exposure (1). Such isotopes are clinically useful in the evaluation of a number of hemodynamic parameters including ventricular ejection fraction and intracardiac shunts as well as evaluation of cardiovascular anatomy.

A number of generator systems have been developed to produce ultrashort-lived isotopes for these applications including Hg-195m/Au-195m, Rb-81/Kr-81m, Cd-109/Ag-109m, and Os-191/Ir-191m. The Os-191/Ir-191m generator has a number of advantages over other systems including high photon yield (>90%), long parent half-life ($T_{1/2}$=15.4d), and the absence of branching pathways. The disadvantage most often cited against the Os-191/Ir-191m generator is the short half-life of the daughter isotope (4.96 s). This is not a disadvantage if a generator of sufficiently high yield could be produced since the short half-life leads to a lower patient radiation dose and a shorter replenish-

0097-6156/84/0241-0051$06.00/0
© 1984 American Chemical Society

ment time for the generator between elutions. For these reasons, we have directed our efforts towards the development of a generator for Ir-191m that has higher yield and lower Os-191 breakthrough than the current design.

Production of Os-191

Os-191 is produced by neutron irradiation of isotopically enriched Os-190 (isotopic composition: Os-190, 97.8%; Os-188, 0.47%; Os-192, 1.02%). Irradiations are currrently performed at the Oak Ridge National Laboratory in the High Flux Isotope Reactor (HFIR) at a neutron flux of 2.5×10^{15} n/cm^2-s. The routes to the various nuclides produced during irradiation of the Os-190 target and the neutron cross-section values (2) are summarized below (Scheme I).

Scheme I. Production scheme for Os-191.

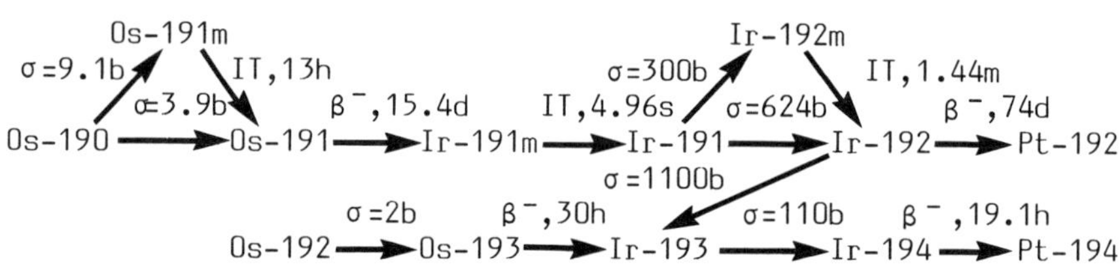

The distribution of the product radionuclides was studied as a function of irradiation periods of from 2-14 days (Table I). These data show that irradiation periods of greater than three or four days do not result in large increases in Os-191 yield but do lead to rapid increases in the Os-193, Ir-192, and Ir-194 impurities. As a result, a three day irradiation period has been chosen as a compromise between Os-191 yield and increasing levels of isotopic impurities. The rapid approach of Os-191 yield to a maximum value during a 14-day irradiation period suggests a maximum attainable specific activity of approximately 600 mCi/mg of enriched Os-190 target.

Examination of Scheme I shows that the principal route to Os-191 is through the formation and subsequent decay of Os-191m ($T_{1/2}$=13h). The total yield is thus the sum of the Os-191 produced by direct neutron capture by Os-190 and from decay of Os-191m. As a result, the maximum Os-191 yield occurs several hours after removal of Os-190 target from the reactor when the Os-191m has decayed to Os-191. With increasing irradiation

Table I . Radionuclides Produced per Milligram of 97.8% Enriched Osmium-190

Irradiation time, days	^{191}Os, mCi	(max)[a]	^{193}Os, mCi	^{192}Ir, mCi	^{194}Ir, mCi
2	170	(45h)	3.6	0.14	...
3	248	(38h)	5.0	0.4	0.4
4	308	(35h)	6.6	0.9	1.0
6	400	(30h)	7.1	2.4	3.4
10	510	(25h)	8.3	5.4	16.5
14	552	(20h)	10.7	7.5	35.0

[a] Hours of target decay following neurtron irradiation required to attain the maximum ^{191}Os value due to a delayed formation by ^{191m}Os decay ($T_{1/2}$=13h).

periods, the time required to achieve maximum Os-191 yield after target removal decreases since the Os-191m level becomes saturated when the rate of production equals the rate of decay. The level of Os-191 continues to increase, however, due to the considerably longer half-life.

A second consequence of increasing irradiation periods is increasing levels of Ir-192 ($T_{1/2}$=74.2d) produced by neutron capture of Ir-191 (Scheme I), which has been formed by decay of the short-lived Ir-191m, the daughter of Os-191. It can be seen from Table I that, for irradiation periods of greater than approximately four days, the amount of Ir-192 increases much more rapidly than that of Os-191. The Ir-192 concentration is a concern because the presence of a significant amount of long-lived Ir-192 in the generator eluate would significantly increase the radiation dose to the patient. The levels of Ir-192 present in these targets have not been found to be a significant problem, however, because they are readily removed by washing the generator with the 4N HCl after loading. Radioassay of the generator eluate after successive washings shows the Ir-192 rapidly decrease to negligible levels while little Os-191 is lost.

The feasibility of producing Os-191 by irradiation of a natural (non-isotopically enriched) osmium target (26.4% Os-190) has also been investigated. A high purity osmium metal target was irradiated in the HFIR at the same neutron flux as the enriched target for 14 days, processed in the usual way, and the radionuclide composition determined by gamma spectrometry. The results show, as expected, a wider range of products are produced than from the isotopically enriched target (3). As in the enriched target, a larger amount of Ir-192 is formed from the increasing amounts of Ir-191 present during prolonged irradiation. In addition, the presence of a greater amount of Os-192 in the target leads to the production of Ir-194 via a similar route (Scheme I). As in the case of the enriched target, both Ir-192 and Ir-194 may be removed by an appropriate rinsing of the generator with 4N HCl prior to use. The other major radiocontaminants present are Os-193 and Os-185. The level of Os-193 may be reduced by decay because of the relatively short half-life (30.5h). The presence of significant amounts of Os-185 is of more concern, despite the low natural abundance of Os-184 in the target mixture. The long half-life ($T_{1/2}$=94d) and the high gamma energies (592 KeV, 1.32%; 646 keV, 80.2%; 717 keV, 4.08%; 875 keV, 6.54%) lead to increased generator shielding requirements and would increase absorbed radiation dose to the patient if there were to be breakthrough of Os-185. This would result in an increased absorbed radiation dose to the patient of approximately 10% compared to that received using a generator prepared from the enriched target material. These results illustrate that, although a satisfactory generator may be prepared from a natural osmium target, the highly enriched Os-190 target material is preferable both for the lower patient radiation dose incurred due to the absence of Os-185 and the elimination of the long decay period prior to generator loading that is required to reduce Os-193 contamination to an acceptable level.

The chemistry of the current generator design requires addition of carrier osmium to the irradiated material to produce a satisfactory generator. This requirement obviates the need for carrier-free Os-191 in the current generator design. Potential sources of carrier-free Os-191 have, however, been surveyed in anticipation of improved generator design. Some potential sources include cycloton production via the Ir-193(d,α)Os-191 reaction; linear accelerator production via the Ir-193 (p,p2n)Os-191 reaction; and spallation of lead with high energy protons, Pb(p,spal)Os-191.

Generator Assembly

Although the procedure for assembly of the Os-191/Ir-191m generator has been previously described (4) several laboratories have reported difficulty in reproducing the results obtained in that study. Recent studies in our laboratory have demonstrated that these difficulties probably result from incomplete description of the generator assembly procedure. We have, therefore, investigated each of these steps and developed a procedure that routinely provides clinically useful generators with 10-15% Ir-191m yield and 5 x 10^{-3}% Os-191 breakthrough (yield and breakthrough are expressed as percent of total Os-191 activity on the column unless otherwise noted).

Preparation of the column. The generator is prepared from a

Lucite tube 1/2" o.d., 3/16" i.d., 3" long (2-1/8" effective column length) equipped with 1/4" x 28 chromatographic fittings. The column has a capacity of approximately 1 ml of anion exchange resin. The AG MP-1 anion exchange resin (100-200 mesh, Cl^- form) is washed successively with distilled water, 0.1N HCl and pH 1 saline and loaded into the Lucite column. The resin is retained within the tube by plastic washers and glass wool at each end of the column. Connections to a luer fitting at each end of the column are made with 1/16" teflon tubing (0.8mm i.d.)

A second (scavenger) column is prepared in the same manner as the main column except that Dowex-2 (200-400 mesh, Cl^- form) is used instead of AG MP-1. In addition the purified Dowex-2 resin is treated by equilibration with catechol (10mg/g resin) in saline at pH 1. The scavenger column is necessary to reduce Os-191 breakthrough to a clinically acceptable level. Both columns are then rinsed with 30 ml of pH 1 saline before use.

Chemical Preparation. The enriched osmium metal target is oxidized by fusion with KNO_3 and KOH for two hours at 500° C. The resulting fusate cake ($K_2[OsO_4(OH)_2]$) is then dissolved in water. A similiar process is carried out with carrier osmium to provide a working solution of 7mg Os/ml. The required amount of irradiated osmium is then combined with enough non-irradiated osmium to give a total of 70 mg. To this solution two pellets (0.2 g) of KOH are added and, after the KOH has dissolved, 35 ml of absolute ethanol is added. A purple precipitate of potassium osmate, $[K_2(OsO_2(OH)_4]$, forms and is isolated by centrifugation and decantation of the excess ethanol. Addition of 4N hydrochloric acid (5ml) to the purple precipitate causes the formation of a brown solution of chloroosmate complexes (primarily $[OsO_2Cl_4]^{2-}$ and $[OsO_2Cl_3(H_2O)]^-$ which is loaded on the anion exchange column.

Loading the generator. The brown chloroosmate solution (prepared as described above) is quickly (<5 min) loaded on the main (AG MP-1) column and the centrifuge tube, transfer pipet, and column rinsed with 1ml 4N HCl. The column is then flushed with air and allowed to equilibrate overnight. The column is rinsed with four 1/2 ml portions of 4N HCl to remove Ir-192, the Dowex-2 scavenger column is attached, and the completed generator rinsed with 30 ml of pH 1 saline. At this stage the Ir-191m yield of the system is 10-15% and the Os-191 breakthrough is 20-80 x 10^{-3}%. The generator is allowed to equilibrate for 24 hours (in pH 1 saline) during which time the breakthrough decreases to 3-5 x 10^{-3}%.

The large number of steps involved in the assembly of this generator and the variability in generator performance arising from small changes in these procedures imply that a significant improvement in performance might be realized from a systematic examination of this system. We have, therefore, studied the effect on yield and breakthrough of a number of changes in the Cheng generator design (4).

Generator Improvements

Main Column. One of the first variables examined was the choice of anion exchange resin. Several commercially available resins were evaluated to determine if one might give rise to a better generator than that prepared with AG MP-1. Data for several

Table II. Effect of Different Resins on Generator Performance

Resin	Yield[a]	Breakthrough[a]
AG MP-1 (100-200 mesh, Cl^-)	1.00	1.00
Dowex 2-X8 (200-400 mesh, Cl^-)	0.44	0.76
AG3-X8 (200-400 mesh, Cl^-)	0.07	1.06
Bio-Rex 9 (200-400 mesh, Cl^-)	3.49	1.35
Dowex 2-X10 (100-200 mesh, Cl^-)	0.65	0.47
Bio-Rex 5 (100-200 mesh, Cl^-)	0.06	0.23

[a] Yield and breakthrough are expressed as ratios of the values for the new resin to that of the standard AG MP-1 system.

of these resins are summarized in Table II. In addition to organic anion exchange resins, a number of inorganic ion exchange materials were examined to determine if these provided higher Ir-191m yield and lower Os-191 breakthrough. The materials examined included zirconium phosphate, alumina, lead sulfide, titanium dioxide, zirconium oxide and stannic oxide but none were observed to retain Os-191 and release Ir-191m.

To evaluate the effects of generator column geometry, a pair of generators were prepared in which the first had the usual dimensions and the second had a main column aproximately 2/3 as long. The amount of osmium metal was reduced to compensate for the smaller volume of the second generator. As may be expected, because of the lower dead volume, the Ir-191m yield of the smaller generator was approximately 50% greater than that of the standard generator. The Os-191 breakthrough of the smaller generator increased by an equivalent amount, however, with no net improvement in performance.

A number of generators were prepared using varying amounts of added "carrier" osmium metal to determine the effect of the total amount of osmium metal on the yield and breakthrough. The yield was found to increase with increasing amounts of osmium loaded on the generator but, unfortunately, the breakthrough increased at approximately the same rate.

Since the distribution of the chlorooxo-osmate species present in the hydrochloric acid solution that is loaded on the generator is affected by the acid concentration (5), a series of generators were prepared using a range of hydrochloric acid concentrations to dissolve the potassium osmate precipitate. The results obtained with these generators are included in Table III. As can be seen from these data, the performance of the

Table III. Effect Of Hydrochloric Acid Concentration[a]

[HCl],N	Yield(%)	Breakthrough(%)
1	5.2	3.8×10^{-3}
2	6.0	4.0×10^{-3}
4	6.0	4.0×10^{-3}
6	6.0	4.8×10^{-3}

[a] Generators eluted with pH 1 saline.

generator is relatively insensitive to such changes in acid concentration. This implies that the species being absorbed on the ion exchange resin is equally well supplied regardless of the initial concentrations of the two predominant osmium complexes, $[OsO_2Cl_4]^{2-}$ and $[OsO_2Cl_3(H_2O)]^{1-}$. These results also imply that the formation of hexachloroosmate(IV) is not a factor as this complex is not present in significant amounts in 1N HCl in the absence of a co-reductant (5).

Scavenger Column. A variety of approaches have also been used in an attempt to increase the effectiveness of the scavenger column. These studies have included varying the size of the scavenger column (and thus the amount of resin available), changing the resin type used in the scavenger column, and using chelating ligands other than catechol. To determine if Os-191 breakthrough could be effectively reduced by increasing the amount of resin used on the scavenger column, a series of generators was prepared coupled with scavenger columns of different geometries. The results of these experiments (Table IV) show that, although the amount of Os-191 breakthrough is decreased with increasing size of the scavenger column, the Ir-191m yield is decreased by a proportionate amount. The net result is that the amount of

Table IV. Effect of Scavenger Column Size on Yield and Breakthrough

Column	Dimensions(l x d,vol.)	Yield(%)	Breakthrough(%)
1	2 1/4" x 3/16",1.0 ml	8.5	26×10^{-3}
2	2 5/8" x 3/16",1.2 ml	6.6	13×10^{-3}
3	2 5/8" x 1/4", 2.2 ml	4.9	9×10^{-3}

(AG2-X10, 100-200 mesh, Cl^- form)

Os-191 injected is not decreased for a given dose of Ir-191m. In addition, the larger column volume increases the dead volume of the generator system and thus increases the volume of eluent required to remove the Ir-191m.

The effect of the addition of various ligands, including catechol, was compared by preparing four identical scavenger columns, each treated with 10 mg of the ligand under study. In addition, a scavenger column prepared with no added ligand and an AG MP-1 column treated with catechol and used as a scavenger column were included. The results of this study are summarized in Table V. From these data, a number of observations were

Table V. Effect of Various Ligands on Generator Yield and Breakthrough

Column	Resin[a]/Ligand	Yield(%)	Breakthrough(%)
1	AG2-X10/catechol	11	6×10^{-3}
2	AG2-X10/ - -	15	8×10^{-3}
3	AG MP-1/catechol	3.2	4×10^{-3}
4	AG2-X10/tropolone	11	5×10^{-3}
5	AG2-X10/8-hydroxyquinoline	10	4×10^{-3}
6	AG2-X10/2,4-pentanedione	10	4×10^{-3}

[a] All resins 100-200 mesh, Cl^-.

made. First, although the addition of catechol decreases the breakthrough by approximately 25% versus that of an untreated column, it also reduces the yield by approximately the same amount, i.e., there is no significant selectivity for osmium versus iridium. A second observation is that, within the limits of experimental error, there is little difference between the performance of scavenger columns prepared with any of the four ligands. Although the ligands are chemically similar, the similar behavior of scavenger columns prepared with these different species is quite interesting. The greatest decrease in breakthrough was observed when the AG MP-1 column was treated with catechol. These results appear to indicate a preference for iridium to osmium in comparison with the AG2-X10/ catechol system. Unfortunately, however, none of these alternative systems show a great enough improvement in either Ir-191m yield or Os-191 breakthrough to justify further evaluation.

Other Changes. Composition of the eluent used with the generator and the effect of pH on yield and breakthrough have been previously discussed by Cheng (4). It was observed that increasing the hydrochloric acid concentration (from the pH 1 saline normally used) increased the Ir-191m yield while the breakthrough remained constant or decreased slightly. Conversely, decreasing the amount of hydrochloric acid (increasing pH) decreased yield and increased breakthrough. In addition, the affect of changing the saline concentration was studied. These data followed a pattern similar to that observed for changes in hydrochloric acid concentration. The choice of eluent is severely limited, however, by the requirement that the injectate be close to physiologic pH and not so hypertonic as to injure the patient. These restrictions effectively limit the pH to no less than 1 while restricting the use of more concentrated sodium chloride solution.

The differences in generator performances resulting from the above changes in the eluent led to the evaluation of a number of possible compounds as additives to the usual pH 1 saline or as substitutes for the hydrochloric acid in the solution. The results of these experiments are summarized in Table VI. These data show that all of these alternative systems, with the exception of 0.254 M hydrochloric acid and 5% ETOH in pH 1 saline, result in a dramatic decrease in the amount of Ir-191m obtained from the generator. The decreased yield is usually accompanied by a decrease in breakthrough. The difficulties of increased acid concentration have been discussed above while the decrease in breakthrough of the ethanol system (17%) is not enough to offset the 13% decrease in yield, particularly in a system where the yield is already low.

In addition to the different eluents, a variety of solutions were evaluated for treatment of the generator after loading. The materials chosen were generally oxidants and reductants on the assumption that the yield and/or breakthrough would be improved if the iridium or osmium could be brought to a more tractable oxidation state. Catechol was included because of its earlier

Table VI. Different Eluents for the Os/Ir Generator

Eluent	Yield(%)[a]	Breakthrough(%)[a]
pH 1 saline	1.00	1.00
HCl (0.254M)	0.72	1.33
pH 1 saline, 5% EtOH	0.87	0.83
citric acid (0.1M)	0.13	0.05
ascorbic acid (0.1M)	<0.01	0.21
edta (0.01M)	0.54	43
acetic acid (0.1M)	0.03	0.93
Na-acetate (0.1M)	<0.01	0.02

[a] Yield and breakthrough are expressed as ratios of values for the test system to the standard generator.

oxidation state. Catechol was included because of its earlier described properties (4) in improving the performance of the generator. The results obtained from this series of experiments are summarized in Table VII. In all cases, the generators

Table VII. Effect of Additions to pH 1 Saline Wash

Wash Solution	Yield (%)[a]	Breakthrough (%)[a]
pH 1 saline, 0.1% ascorbic acid	0.90	31.
" 0.1% H_2O_2	0.31	65.
" 0.1% $SnCl_2$	1.00	250.
" 0.1% catechol	0.82	0.50
" 0.01% catechol	1.10	0.70
" 0.5% catechol	0.35	0.38

[a] Yield and breakthrough are expressed as ratios of values for test system to those of the standard generator. Generators eluted with pH 1 saline.

were flushed with 30 ml of the test solution and then eluted with standard pH 1 saline. The first of these solutions, ascorbic acid, hydrogen peroxide, and stannous chloride had the opposite of the desired effect, increasing breakthrough without increasing yield. Treatment of the generator with 0.01% catechol in pH 1 saline was found to decrease breakthrough significantly (30%) and, at the same time, modestly (10%) increase Ir-191m yield.

In summary, despite the evaluation of a wide variety of possible changes in the current generator design, none, with the exception of pretreatment with 0.01% catechol in pH 1 saline, were found to result in significant improvements in the performance of the generator. Although we now routinely treat generators with catechol, the yield is still about 10-15%, which is less than optimal. As a result, our recent efforts have been directed towards the development of a new generator design rather than improvements in the current generator.

New Generator Designs

The search for a new generator design has been directed towards the evaluation of chemical systems that might offer a combination of ease of preparation and chemical stability. To be useful in clinical evaluations the chemistry of the generator system must be straightforward since elaborate synthetic facilities are not generally available in clinical departments. The interest in increased chemical stability arises from the problems encountered with the current generator design and the observation that the complex changes color from light brown to black after absorption on the AG MP-1 resin. It has been suggested that the breakthrough arises, at least partially, from decomposition of the parent Os complex on the strongly basic anion exchange resin (4). Our early attempts to circumvent these problems made use of two readily prepared osmate complexes; trans-dioxotetrahydroxoosmate(VI), $[OsO_2(OH)_4]^{2-}$, and trans-dioxotetracyanoosmate(VI), $[OsO_2(CN)_4]^{2-}$.

trans-Dioxotetrahydroxoosmate(VI) is prepared by ethanol reduction of potassium perosmate, as described above. In this case, however, the resulting purple precipitate is dissolved in distilled water rather than 4N hydrochloric acid. Generators prepared with this complex exhibited low Os-191 breakthrough but, unfortunately, the Ir-191m yield was also low. The complex was found to be unstable both in water and when absorbed on the anion exchange resin.

trans-Dioxotetracyanoosmate(VI) is prepared by addition of KCN to an aqueous solution of either $[OsO_2(OH)_4]^{2-}$ or $[OsO_4(OH)_2]^{2-}$ and has been reported to be quite stable (6). A generator was prepared by absorption of this complex on AG MP-1 anion exchange resin. When eluted with saline the yield of this generator was 10-15% while the breakthrough was 5×10^{-3}%, approximately the same as the current design. The use of an eluent consisting of 0.01M KCN/0.154M saline caused a small decrease in breakthrough but a large decrease in yield. Although the use of saline in this generator is obviously preferable to the acid eluent used in the Cheng generator design, the presence of cyanide in the system with no improvement in performance mitigates against further efforts with this system.

The poor performance of these systems led to consideration of osmium complexes that might better stabilize the trans-dioxo-osmate(VI) moiety and, perhaps, at the same time stabilize the resulting iridium complex, allowing it to be more readily eluted and thereby increasing the yield. A second consideration is that the overall -2 charge of the complex should be maintained so that the complexes will be tightly retained on anion exchange resins. A number of ligands were evaluated including, ethylenediamine-tetraacetic acid (edta), citric acid, ascorbic acid, oxalic acid, malonic acid, and catechol. Generators were prepared using each of these ligands in place of the usual 4N HCl and the yield and breakthrough measured. Based on this screening the most promising system utilized malonic acid. Our recent efforts have, therefore, been directed towards maximizing the performance of this system.

The eluent solution of the generator was examined to determine the affect of added malonic acid, pH, and saline concentrations. The yield and breakthrough were maximized with an eluent consisting of 0.05M malonic acid, 0.10M saline at pH 4, a slightly hypertonic mixture. With this eluent, an Ir-191m yield of 30-35% was obtained with an Os-191 breakthrough of 3×10^{-3}%. In comparison, these values are approximately twice as good as those routinely obtained with the standard Cheng generator both in terms of yield and breakthrough. In the clinical setting this would correspond to a four-fold decrease in the amount of osmium injected per millicurie of iridium-191m with a corresponding decrease in the patient radiation dose. In addition, these generators are relatively insensitive to the amount of osmium metal loaded, require no scavenger column to achieve this low breakthrough, and buffering of the eluate prior to injection is not necessary.

A disadvantage of this generator system, however, is the fact that the yield (expressed as a percentage of loaded osmium activity) decreases at a more rapid rate (approximately 5%/day) than that observed with the $[OsO_2Cl_4]^{2-}$ system (Table VIII). The net result is that after four days the generator has approximately the same elution characteristics as the Cheng generator. After this time, however, the yield is less than that of the Cheng design while the breakthrough remains at the same low level. A number of approaches have been attempted unsuccessfully to stabilize the generator. The rapid decrease in yield is at least partially offset by the fact that on the day after assembly the generator may be used clinically whereas the earlier design must be allowed to equilibrate for another day before the breakthrough decreases sufficiently for clinical use. The combination of increased yield, decreased breakthrough, absence of a scavenger column, and "bufferless" eluent make this the most promising system found thus far and preliminary evaluation of this system in laboratory animals is currently underway.

Table VIII. Elution Performance of Malonic Acid vs. Chloro Generator With Time[a]

	H_2mal		HCl	
Date	Yield(%)	Break-through(%)	Yield(%)	Break-through(%)
4/12	30	4.4×10^{-3}	14	11×10^{-3}
4/13	24	2.8×10^{-3}	15	5.8×10^{-3}
4/14	20	2.9×10^{-3}	14	5.6×10^{-3}
4/15	14	2.8×10^{-3}	13	4.2×10^{-3}

[a] Generator assembled and loaded 4/11.

Clinical Applications

The Os-191/Ir-191m generator has been used clinically at Children's Hospital for several years and the use of Ir-191m for first-pass radionuclide angiography for the detection and quantitation of shunts and the evaluation of cardiac function has been discussed (1,7,8). In pediatric patients, the primary application of this technique has been the detection and quantitation of intracardiac shunts. Figure 1 shows the results of a study in a 2 year-old female patient. The radionuclide can be seen entering the heart via an intracardiac catheter, passing through the right heart, the lungs, and finally the left heart. Figure 2 shows the pulmonary time-activity curve obtained from the right lung of the same patient. The curve has been corrected for count loss due to camera dead-time and for radioactive decay. The Qp:Qs value has been determined by the method of Maltz and Treves (9) and reveals extensive early recirculation due to left-to-right shunting (region B).

Cardiac function may be evaluated by the determination of left (or right) ventricular ejection fraction (VEF). In this procedure, regions of interest are defined at the end diastolic and end systolic phases of heart beat. The ejection fraction is defined as the ratio of tracer (blood) in the heart in the contracted (systolic) versus the relaxed (diastolic) phases of the heart cycle with appropriate corrections for decay and gamma camera dead time. The value obtained provides a measure of the ability of the heart to pump blood through the lungs (RVEF) or the body (LVEF). A criticism of Ir-191m for this application has been that the half-life (4.96s) is too short to allow effective visualization and quantitation of left ventricular function in adults, particularly those with delayed transit times. A recent

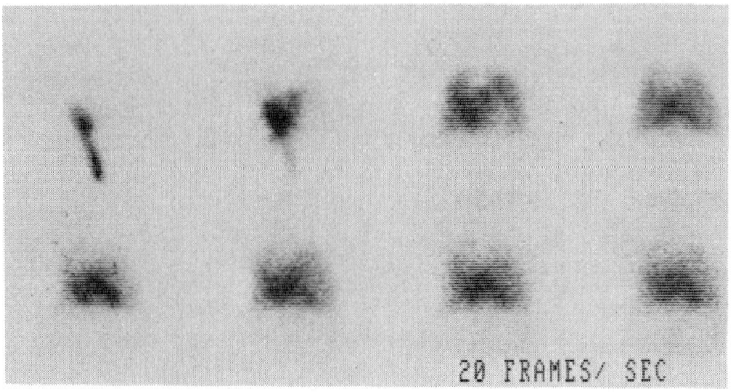

Figure 1. Radionuclide angiogram recorded with Ir-191m.

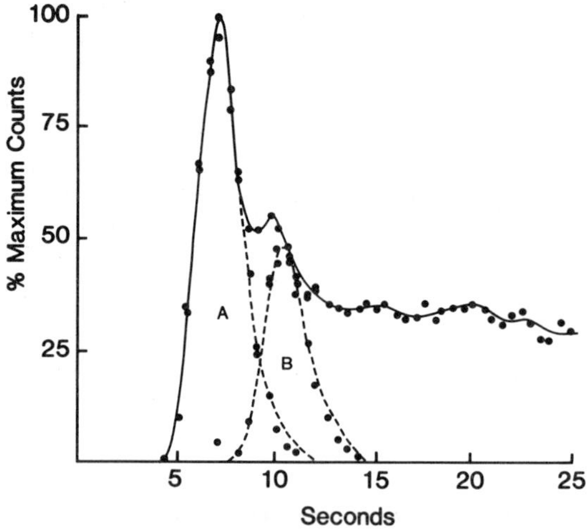

Figure 2. Deconvoluted time-activity curve of right lung of patient in Figure 1. Secondary curves are least squares fits from which the Qp:Qs values are derived. Region A - normal pulmonary perfusion. Region B - early recirculation due to left-to-right shunt.

study, in collaboration with workers at Beth Israel Hospital, has demonstrated, however, that sufficient activity is present in the left ventricle for effective measurement (10). In addition, recent studies at Children's Hospital in young adults with cor pulmonale due to cystic fibrosis have shown that both LVEF and RVEF decrease in response to submaximal exercise (11). In this same study, comparison of VEF values obtained with Ir-191m to those obtained with Tc-99m showed equivalent results.

Other current applications of Ir-191m angiography include diagnosis of congenital circulatory defects (i.e., tetrology of Fallot) and vena caval obstruction. Potential applications that remain to be explored include measurement of ventricular volume, renal perfusion, cerebral blood flow, and evaluation of blood flow to tumors and organs by selective arterial infusion.

Summary

The use of Ir-191m in pediatric radionuclide angiography for the quantitation of shunts and ejection fraction and the diagnosis of a variety of congentital cardiovascular malformations is well established. Preliminary results suggest that the determination of LVEF is also possible in adults using Ir-191m but a more complete study is needed to compare these results with those obtained using Tc-99m. In addition, a variety of potential applications (described above) have yet to be fully explored.

Although the generator currently in clinical use has proven adequate for feasibility studies, a simpler design that provides both higher Ir-191m yield and lower Os-191 breakthrough is needed before the use of the generator can be fully explored with more widespread clinical trials. The malonate design described in this paper is a step in that direction and clearly demonstrates that an Os-191/Ir-191m generator with both higher yield and lower breakthrough is possible. Our current efforts are directed towards application of the chemical data acquired to date to produce a generator with still higher yield and sufficient stability to more fully exploit the long half-life of the parent isotope.

Acknowledgments

This work was supported by the U.S.D.O.E. Contract #DE-AC02-82ER60084 and the Fanny Ripple Foundation. Work at the Oak Ridge National Laboratory was supported by the Office of Health and Environmental Research, U.S. Department of Energy, under contract W-7405-eng-26 with the Union Carbide Corporation.

Literature Cited

1. Treves, S.; Cheng, C., Samuel, A.; Lambrecht, R.; Babchyck, B.; Zimmerman, R.; Norwood, W. J. Nucl. Med. 1980, 21, 1151-1157.

2. Mughabghab, S.F.; Garber, D.I. "Neutron Cross Sections"; Vol. 1, Resonance Parameters, BNL 325, Third Edition, Brookhaven National Laboratory; Uptown, NY, 1973.
3. Butler, T.A., Guyer, C.E., Knapp, F.F. Jr. Proceedings Third World Congress of Nuclear Medicine and Biology. 1982, 617-620.
4. Cheng, C.; Treves, S.; Samuel, A.; Davis, M.A. J. Nucl. Med. 1980, 21, 1169-1176.
5. Bremard, C.; Mouchel, B. Inorg. Chem. 1982, 21, 1810.
6. Krauss, F.; Schrader, G. J. Prakt. Chem. 1929, 120, 36.
7. Treves, S.; Kulprathipanja, S.; Hnatowich, D.J. Circulation 1976, 54, 275-279.
8. Kulprathipanja, S.; Hnatowich, D.J.; Davis, M.A.; Treves, S. in "Medical Radionuclide Imaging"; IAEA: Vienna, 1977; Vol. II, pp. 53-59.
9. Maltz, D.L.; Treves, S. Circulation 1973, 47, 1049-1056.
10. Heller, G., personal communication.
11. Dozier, A., personal communication.

RECEIVED October 14, 1983

A Rb-81/Kr-81m Perfusion Generator

M. S. PHILP, C. I. RAMSEY, J. M. MA, and J. F. LAMB

Medi-Physics, Inc., 5801 Christie Avenue, Emeryville, CA 94608

A Rb-81/Kr-81m perfusion generator is under development at Medi-Physics, Inc. The generator consists of a glass column with a glass filter disc filled with approximately 200 mg wet cation exchange resin. The Rb-81 solution is loaded onto the column in a single pass with greater than 95% efficiency. The Kr-81m is eluted with greater than 85% efficiency in non-ionic dextrose solution and administered I.V. Rubidium-81 washoff from the generator during elution varies with flow rate and total eluate volume, but remains less than 5 µCi per 100 cc eluate.

Krypton-81m has been used to study cardiopulmonary systems from as early as 1970 (1,2). Since then other investigators have proposed its use for myocardial perfusion, (3,4), cerebral perfusion, (5,6), and venography, (7). A Rb-81/Kr-81m generator for pulmonary ventilation studies has been commercially available since 1980 from Medi-Physics, Inc. The present work will focus on the manufacture and testing of a Rb-81/Kr-81m generator suitable for liquid elution and use in perfusion studies.

Experimental

The parent nuclide, Rb-81, is produced by proton bombardment of a krypton gas target enriched in Kr-82 to about 70%. Usual bombardment conditions are 22 Mev protons at 40-45 microamps. Typical yields of Rb-81 are 12 to 15 mCi/µAh at end of bombardment, with 15 to 17% Rb-82m produced from the (p,n) reaction. Since Rb-82m decays to stable Kr-82, it does not contribute any impurities to the generator eluate. The radioisotopes of rubidium produced during bombardment are rinsed from the target with sterile water. Samples of the target solution are assayed for Rb-81, and volumes of solution containing 5, 10, or 20 mCi are dispensed into sterile sealed vials. The Kr-81m generators are assembled from sterile components and placed in lead shields. The generator consists of

0097-6156/84/0241-0067$06.00/0
© 1984 American Chemical Society

a small glass tube with a sintered glass filter at one end and filled with approximately 200 mg moist cation exchanger. The glass column is 35-40 mm long with an I.D. of 4 mm; 15 to 20 mm is filled with the resin. The cation exchange resin is Bio Rad AG MP-50, a macroporous styrene divinyl benzene polymer with sulfonic acid exchange groups. Small bore, sterile polyvinylchloride connecting tubes are used as inlet and outlet lines. The rubidium radioisotopes are quantitatively absorbed onto the cation resin during a single pass under slight suction. Each generator is then washed with 20 to 50 ml of sterile water. The loading and wash solutions are collected and tested for Rb-81 content, sterility, and endotoxins.

Preliminary performance tests on the generator include an evaluation of the loading efficiency of Rb-81 and the elution efficiency of Kr-81m, an evaluation of the levels of microscopic and particulate matter washed off during elution, and the effect of radioactivity on the cation resin. The loading efficiencies were measured by Ge(Li) spectrometric assay of the 191 keV peak of Kr-81m in an exposed generator column both during elution with 5% dextrose solution and without elution when in equilibrium with Rb-81. Rubidium-81 breakthrough was determined by Ge(Li) assay of Rb-81 in 100 ml of 5% dextrose eluate. Particulate matter washed off during elution was measured via the USP XX procedure (8). The effect of radioactivity on the cation exchange resin was investigated by preparing a 50 mCi generator and eluting with 25 ml water after 36 hours. The eluate was tested by high pressure liquid chromatography (HPLC), gas chromatography (GC), ultraviolet spectroscopy (u.v.), and fluoroscopy with a comparison to a control sample from a nonradioactive generator. The following test conditions were used:

HPLC	Radial PAK C-18 column Methanol eluant at 2 ml/min
GC	Porapak Q column with He carrier gas
u.v.	Bausch & Lomb Spectronic 200 u.v., Scanned from 350-200nm against deionized water
Fluoroscopy	Excitation energy at 360nm Detection energy at 415nm

Results and Discussion

Loading efficiencies were measured for a series of 30 generators ranging in activity from 5 to 20 mCi. In all cases loading efficiencies exceeded 99%. Optimum loading was achieved at flow rates of less than 10 ml/min and resin weights greater than 150 mg (column length greater than 15 mm). Elution of Kr-81m from 24 generators tested averaged 85.9 ± 0.8% at flow rates of 14 to 17 ml/min. At flow rates of less than 10 ml/min the measured elution efficiency dropped to about 80% due to increased transit time across the Ge(Li) detector field of view. The elution efficiency remained constant over the time of use of the generator. The amount of Kr-81m available at the exit of a 6 inch output line from a 10 mCi generator at various flow rates is shown in Table I.

Table I: Kr-81m Available at 6 inch Output Line for Various Eluant Flow Rates from a 10 mCi Generator

Eluant Flow Rate (ml/min)	Available Kr-81m (mCi)
5	5.8
10	6.9
15	7.3
20	7.6

The amount of Rb-81 breakthrough during elution with 5% dextrose solution was measured for 30 generators and varied from 0.5 to 5.0 μCi in 100 ml of eluate, with an average value of 1.2 ± 1.1 μCi. The Rb-81 breakthrough increased with volume of eluant passed through the generator (Figure 1) and with elution flowrate (Figure 2). Washoff of microscopic particulate matter during elution of two generators passed USP XX specifications, however, they were close to the limit for particles greater than 25 μm size. Use of a sterilizing 0.22 μm filter downstream decreased observable particulates to well below specifications. No resin degradation products were detected in the 25 ml eluate from a 50 mCi generator when tested by GC, HPLC, or fluoroscopy. However, some u.v. absorbing material was observed in the u.v. scan (Abs ∿0.1). Subsequent elution of the generator yielded no detectable material.

Summary

Manufacture of Rb-81/Kr-81m generator for use in perfusion studies is relatively simple and straightforward. Elution characteristics are suitable for clinical use. Figure 3 shows a supine image and an upright image of the right heart, pulmonary outflow tract and lungs with the upright image demonstrating the postural shift in blood flow away from the apex of the lungs. This scan was done during a continuous infusion of Kr-81m from a 10 mCi generator.

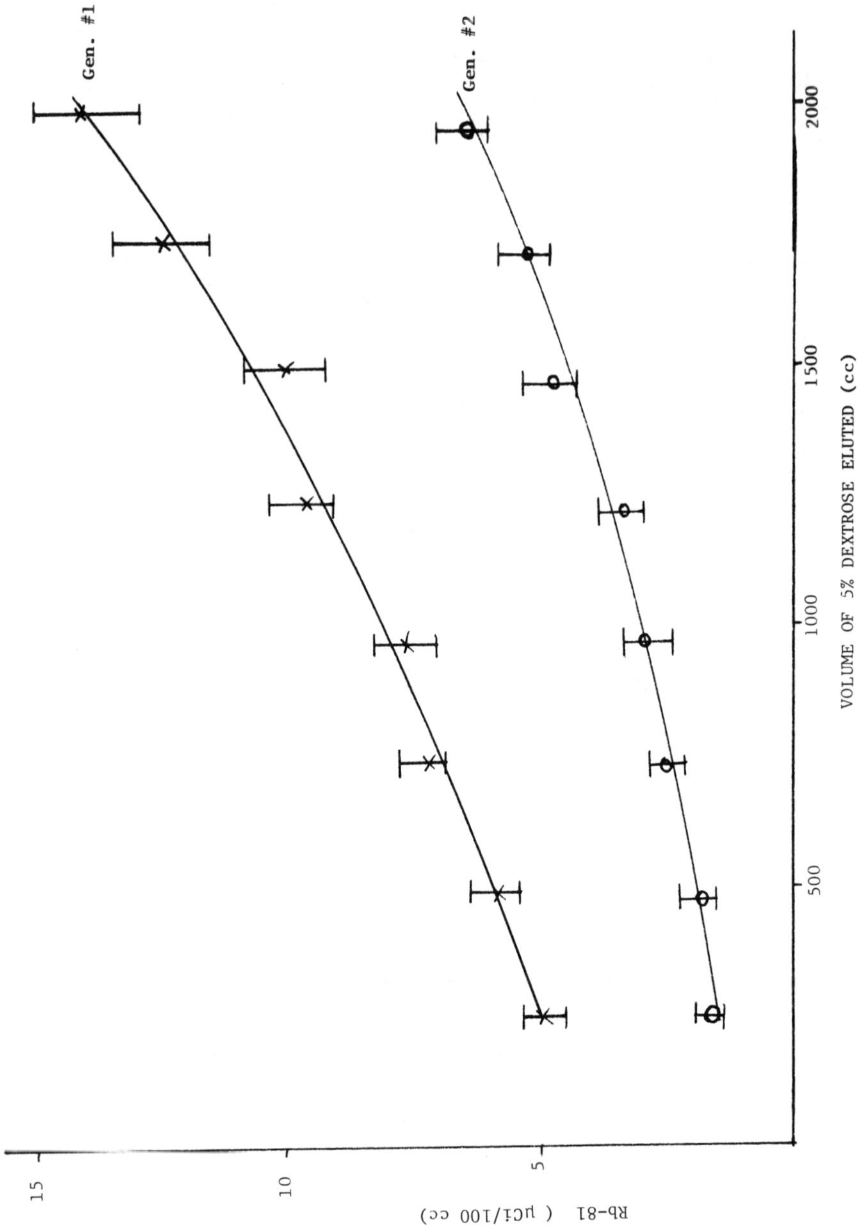

Figure 1. Rb-81 washoff for 2 L 5% dextrose elutions (20mCi generators).

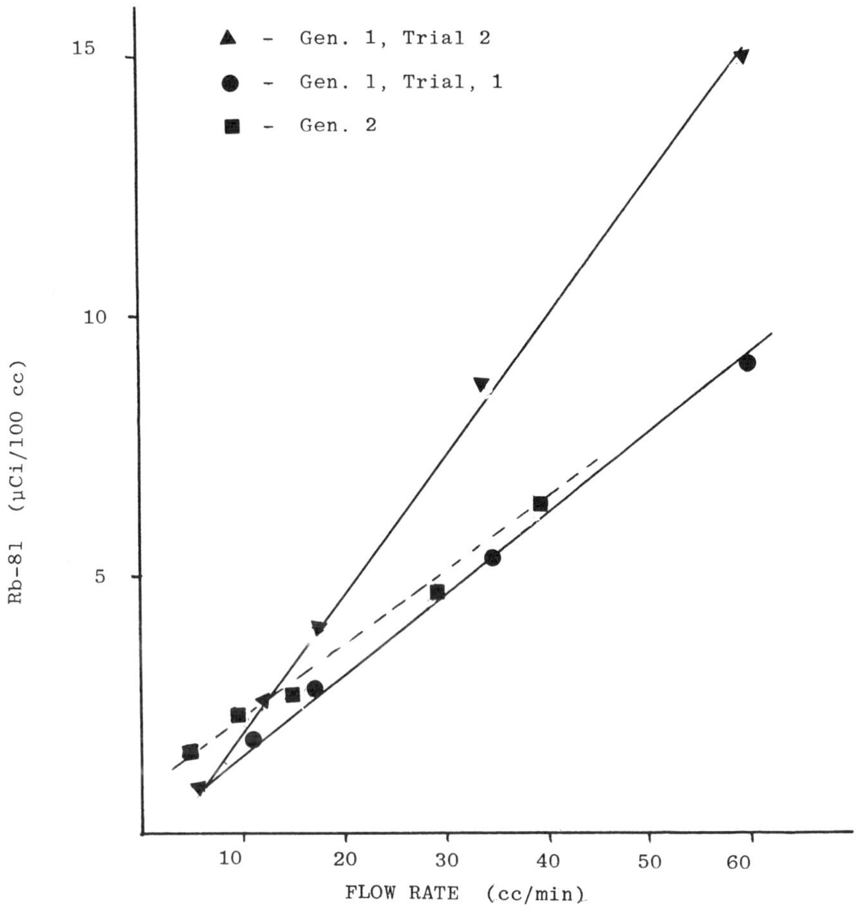

Figure 2. Rb-81 washoff vs. eluant flow rate (20 mCi generators).

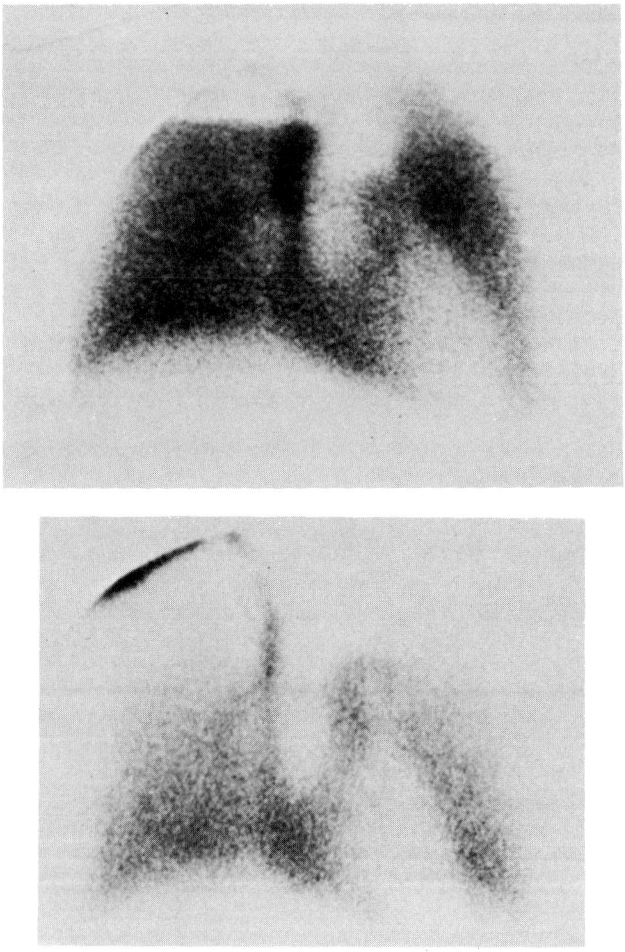

Figure 3. Lung perfusion anterior scan using Kr-81m. Top, supine; bottom, upright. (Photo courtesy of Drs. Matthew Horn and Kathryn Witztum, VA Medical Center, University of California, San Diego.)

Literature Cited

1. Jones, T.; Clark, J.C.; Hughes, J.M.; Rosenwerg, D.Y. J. Nucl. Med., 1970, 11, 118-124.
2. Yano, Y.; McRae, J.; Anger, H.O. J. Nucl. Med., 1970, 11, 674-679.
3. Kaplan, E.; Mayron, L.W.; Friedman, A.M.; Gindler, J.E.; Frazin, L.; Moran, J.M.; Loeb, H.; Gunnar, R.M. Am. J. Card., 1976, 37, 878-884.
4. Turner, J.U.; Selwyn, A.P.; Jones, T.; Evans, T.F.; Raphael, M.U.; Lavendar, J.P. Cardiovasc. Res., 1976, 10, 398-404.
5. Mayron, L.W.; Kaplan, E.; Friedman, A.M.; Gindler, J.E. Int. J. Nucl. Med. Biol., 1976, 3, 35-36.
6. Fazio, F.; Nardini, M.; Fieschi, C.; Forli, C.; J. Nucl. Med., 1977, 18, 962-966.
7. Bassett, L.W.; Bennett, L.R.; Witt, E.; Webber, M.M. Int. J. Nucl. Med. Biol., 1970, 7, 378.
8. "Large Volume in Injections for Single Dose Infusion", U.S. Pharmacopeia, 20th Ed., July 1, 1980, 863.

RECEIVED August 19, 1983

POSITRON-EMITTING RADIONUCLIDES

6

Production of Radionuclides for Generator Systems

LEONARD F. MAUSNER, THOMAS PRACH, and POWELL RICHARDS

Medical Department, Brookhaven National Laboratory, Upton, NY 11973

Recently there has been a significant increase in interest in generator produced short-lived radionuclides. Developments on three short-lived positron-emitting generator systems which can be produced at the Brookhaven LINAC Isotope Producer (BLIP) are described. The Fe-52/Mn-52m positron system is attractive for the study of myocardial perfusion because radiomanganese demonstrates good myocardial uptake with extremely rapid blood clearance resulting in high myocardium-to-blood ratios. The 21 minute half-life of Mn-52m also allows repeat studies to monitor intervention. Our production parameters for this generator are presented. The Xe-122/I-122 combination, a convenient source of a short-lived (3.6m) positron emitting iodine, is also discussed. Recent developments in rapid iodination procedures will broaden the potential applications of this generator. Finally, preliminary investigations of another generator derived radionuclide that may have promise is described. Tellurium-118 (6d) is the parent of the 3.5 minute positron emitter Sb-118 which may be useful for first pass angiography.

The field of nuclear medicine has grown tremendously in the last two decades largely as a result of the development of the Mo-99/Tc-99m generator system. The ready availability of Tc-99m created a mushrooming interest in nuclear medicine clinical and research activity. Technetium-99m in a variety of forms is annually used in millions of nuclear medicine procedures performed worldwide. During recent years there has been a significant increase in interest in very short-lived (<30 min)

0097-6156/84/0241-0077$06.00/0
© 1984 American Chemical Society

radionuclides to maximize photon yield with minimum radiation exposure. The use of short-lived radionuclides offers significantly lower radiation dose to patients, improved studies with high photon flux, the possibility of repeat studies or rapid sequential studies, and the possibility of multiple radionuclide procedures within a short time. In general, the only practical method for widespread distribution of such radionuclides is through generator systems. This article will describe some new generator systems for short-lived positron emitters that are in various stages of development in the radionuclide research program centered on the Brookhaven Linac Isotope Producer (BLIP). The availability of these positron emitters could significantly broaden the potential applications of positron emission tomography.

The generator systems included are Fe-52/Mn-52m, Xe-122/I-122 and Te-118/Sb-118. The iron-manganese system is attractive for the study of myocardial perfusion because radiomanganese demonstrates good myocardial uptake with extremely rapid blood clearance. This quickly results in very favorable myocardium to blood ratios. The 21.1 minute half-life of Mn-52m is short enough to allow repeat studies to monitor the efficacy of therapeutic intervention. Our work with this generator is presented in detail below. The Xe-122/I-122 combination, a convenient source of a short-lived (3.6 m) positron emitting iodine, is also discussed. Recent developments in rapid iodination procedures will increase the usefulness of this generator. Finally, preliminary investigations of an attractive new generator system, Te-118/Sb-118 is described. Tellurium-118 ($t_{1/2}$ = 6 d) is the parent of the 3.5 minute positron emitter Sb-118 which may be useful for first pass angiography.

Fe-52/Mn-52m

Manganese is a necessary trace metal in man and within the cell, much of the manganese is localized in mitochondria. This fact motivated several studies (1,2) of the use of radiomanganese as a tracer for assessment of myocardial perfusion. Studies in rats and dogs indicated favorable ratios of myocardium-to-blood concentration even after very short times following intravenous administration, and myocardial uptake was similar to widely used Tl-201. Manganese-52m is the only nuclide of manganese that has suitable properties for imaging regional myocardial perfusion and the special advantage of availability from a generator (3). It emits annihilation radiation in high abundance (∿1.9 annihilation photons per decay), useful for obtaining high contrast transaxial tomograms. The accompanying 1434 keV gamma rays (97.8% abundance) do not significantly affect coincident detection techniques. The relevant nuclear data of the Fe-52/Mn-52m system are shown in Figure 1.

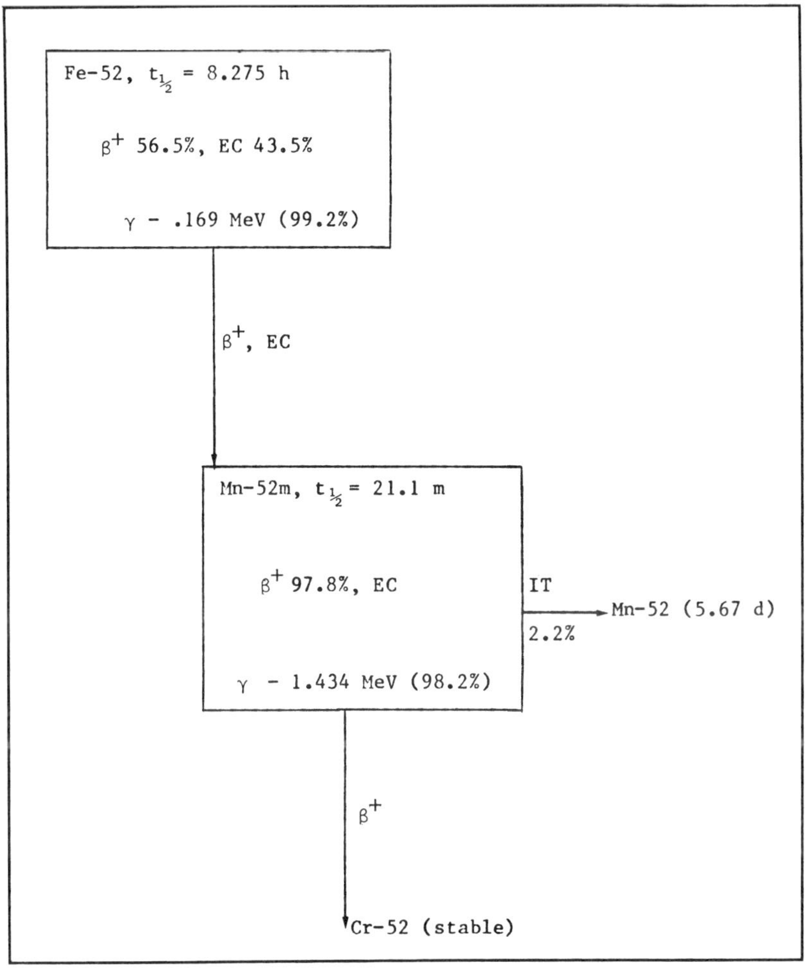

Figure 1. Fe-52/Mn-52m decay characteristics.

Method. Iron-52 ($t_{1/2}$ = 8.275 h) is produced by bombarding a manganese or nickel target at the BLIP (4). The manganese target consists of natural manganese flakes, 2.7 g/cm^2 thick, contained in a capsule formed by a 5 cm (ID) stainless steel ring sealed with 0.25 mm stainless steel windows. Iron-52 is formed by the interaction of 70 MeV protons with manganese by the Mn-55(p,4n) Fe-52 reaction. The nickel target is simply a 0.5 mm nickel foil. Iron-52 is produced in this target with 200 MeV protons, mainly by the (p,3p4n) reaction on Ni-58 (68.3% abundance). Small additional contributions are produced by (p,3pxn) reactions on other nickel isotopes. A typical bombardment lasts for 17 hours at an average beam current of 50 microamperes.

Following irradiation, both the manganese and nickel targets are dissolved in hot 12N nitric acid with a few drops of hydrogen peroxide. For both targets, Fe-52 is separated from the target matrix and other reaction products by means of an anion-exchange method. After adjusting the target solution to 6N in HCl by mixing with concentrated hydrochloric acid, it is sucked through a pretreated ion exchange column (AG 1 x 8, 200-400 mesh resin, Bio-Rad Laboratories, Richmond, CA, 1.8 cm dia. x 2 cm long) at a flow rate of 25 ml/min at 50°C. The column is then washed with two portions of 100 ml of 6N HCl followed by two portions of 65 ml of 4N HCl at 4 ml/min at 80°C. Iron-52 is finally eluted with three 10-ml portions of 0.01N HCl at 80°C under gravity. The Fe-52 recovery is consistently higher than 90%.

The generator column consists of the lower two-thirds of a 1-ml plastic tuberculin syringe barrel filled with 0.6 ml of pretreated anion exchange resin (same as above) supported by a porous disc of inert polypropylene. The Fe-52 solution, or part of it, is transferred to a glass chamber and made 8N in HCl. The solution is subsequently forced by air pressure through the column of the generator in which Fe-52 is adsorbed as $FeCl_4^-$. An additional 5 ml of 8N HCl is run through the generator to wash the column. The entire procedure from the end of the irradiation to this point requires about 2.5 hours.

The generator is eluted with 2 ml of 8N HCl. The eluate is evaporated on a hot plate in a stream of filtered nitrogen gas until dry. The Mn-52m is then redissolved in 3 ml of sodium acetate buffer (pH = 5.6). The solution is passed through a disposable 0.45 μm bacterial filter before injection to ensure sterility of the Mn-52m. These steps take less than 10 minutes.

Results. The Fe-52 production parameters are summarized in Table I. The yields and purity were determined by gamma spectroscopy. Iron-52 from the nickel target contains a trace of 44.6-d Fe-59 impurity (average 0.33% at end of bombardment). The 2.7-y Fe-55 impurity, which emits 5.9-keV (24.3%) and 6.5-keV (3.3%) x-rays and no gamma rays, is determined by means of a high-resolution Si(Li) x-ray detector or thin window Ge detector. It amounts to 0.7% for a manganese target and 0.8% for a nickel target at end of bombardment (EOB). However, when used in a generator, these impurities would present no problem to the radionuclidic quality of Mn-52m since they are retained on the column and their daughters are nonradioactive.

Because of the complexity of the Ni-58(p,3p4n)Fe-52 reaction, the excitation function is expected to show a monotonical rise from the threshold energy and then remain relatively flat once the maximum is reached. Consequently, an increase in nickel target thickness should raise the yield proportionately. The concentrations of Fe-55 and Fe-59 impurities in the product are also expected to remain unchanged for the same reason. This has been qualitatively checked by simultaneously bombarding 4 Ni foils (.023 g/cm^2 each) placed in our target stack such that the incident proton energies were 192, 127, 80 and 61 MeV, respectively. After correction for beam attenuation the yields were essentially constant.

Iron-52 produced in charged-particle accelerators is virtually carrier-free. However, stable iron could be introduced from target materials and reagents or through improper handling. For generator use, high specific activity is necessary in order to minimize column size and reduce Fe-52 breakthrough. In this work, high-purity manganese and nickel, containing less than 10 ppm iron impurity (according to specifications from the manufacturer), are utilized as target materials. Reagent-grade acids are used in the chemical processing. To remove the last traces of stable iron contaminants, the acids are further purified beforehand by passing the HCl through an anion exchange column and by distilling the HNO_3. Dilutions of the acids and solutions are performed with ultrapure water ("Super Q Water" filter system obtained from Millipore Corp., Bedford, MA, with resistance >10 megohms). The amount of iron present in the final Fe-52 solution, as determined by atomic absorption, is of the order of 100-500 µg at end of bombardment. The specific activity is higher than 0.15 mCi/µg at end of bombardment.

A typical elution curve of the Fe-52/Mn-52m generator is shown in Figure 2. Obviously the yield can be somewhat increased with larger elution volumes. However, since this solution must be evaporated for conversion to acetate some compromise is necessary. With the column having a 0.6 ml resin bed, approximately 90% of the generated Mn-52m is recovered in 2 ml of 8N HCl. Figure 3 is a gamma-ray spectrum of the eluted Mn-52m obtained using a Ge(Li) detector coupled to a multichannel analyzer. The radionuclidic impurities were determined after the short-lived Mn-52m had decayed and no Fe-52 breakthrough was detected. An upper limit of 1×10^{-7} of Fe-52 breakthrough was derived from our minimum detectable activity of 0.001 µCi. The only activity found was Mn-52 from the decay of Mn-52m. Manganese-52m decays in two branches; 97.8% goes to stable Cr-52 and 2.2% goes to 5.67-d Mn-52. Decay-growth calculations indicate that 3.2×10^{-4}% of Mn-52 (relative to Mn-52m) is formed

Table I. Fe-52 Production Parameters

Target Material:	Manganese (2.7 g/cm^2)	Nickel (0.45 g/cm^2)
Nuclear Reaction	Mn-55(p,4n)Fe-52	Ni-58(p,3p4n)Fe-52
Ep* (Incident)	70 MeV	193.0 MeV
Ep (Exit)	50 MeV	191.6 MeV
Production Rate	98 μCi/μAh	50 μCi/μAh
Typical Yield (EOB)	60 mCi	33 mCi

*Proton energy

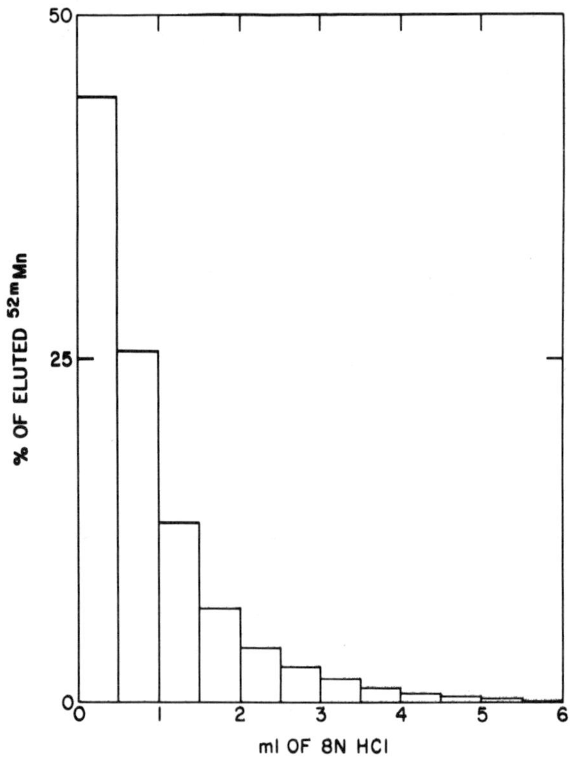

Figure 2. Elution profile of the Mn-52m generator. (Reproduced with permission from Ref. 5. Copyright 1979, Radiological Society of America, Inc.)

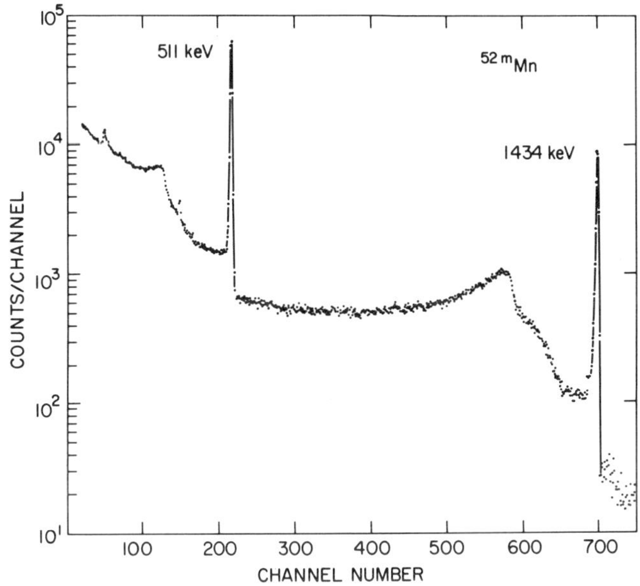

Figure 3. Mn-52m gamma spectrum.

in the generator column in a typical growth period of one hour. Manganese-52 from the decay of Mn-52m at 118 minutes after elution would amount to 5.6 x 10^{-3}% of what the Mn-52m had been at time of elution. The presence of such small amounts would have a negligible impact on the total radiation dose to the patient. This work is also detailed by Ku et al. (5).

The elution yield and iron breakthrough were measured as a function of time and number of elutions. Six elutions were performed over a period of 26 hours and gave essentially constant Mn-52m recovery, averaging 93% of the available radioactivity. No iron breakthrough was observed from these elutions. Utilizing the Fe-59 impurity, breakthrough was checked up to five days after end of bombardment, long past the useful life of the generator. There was still no detectable iron breakthrough. Thus column resin degradation is minimal and the generator can be safely used for as long as practical levels of radioactivity remain.

Animal studies. Distribution data in animals were obtained using Mn-54 for convenience, administered as the chloride and acetate (2). Clearance from the blood was extremely rapid, with a $t_{½}$ of less than one minute in dogs (Figure 4). This resulted in a high myocardium-to-blood concentration ratio. The myocardial uptake in dogs was greater than 3%/organ at three and 15 minutes, with myocardium-to-blood ratios of about 40:1 at 15 minutes. There was good correlation (r = 0.89) between the regional distribution of radiolabeled microspheres and manganese in the normal and infarcted myocardium. Positron tomograms were obtained with Mn-52m eluted from the generator described above. These demonstrated regional myocardial perfusion in a normal dog and clearly visualized a perfusion defect after ligation of the coronary artery. Absorbed radiation dose estimates from Mn-52m were calculated using biodistribution from dogs. The dose for selected organs was (in rad/mCi) whole body 0.032, heart 0.154, blood 0.041, liver 0.291, lungs 0.058, and ovaries 0.068. A subsequent investigation (6) studied the resolution and sensitivity of Mn-52m as a quantitative measurement of the size and location of myocardial ischemia. Comparison between microsphere distributions and Mn-52m images taken at 1.5 cm levels revealed that an ischemic area down to the size of 2.5 cm^2 with 50% of the normal myocardial perfusion can be seen in the positron images. In addition, a relative change of 10% or more of the normal perfusion in the ischemic area can also be observed. Large clinical studies with the Fe-52m/Mn-52m generator have recently been initiated at the National Heart and Lung and Institute, National Institutes of Health, Bethesda, Maryland.

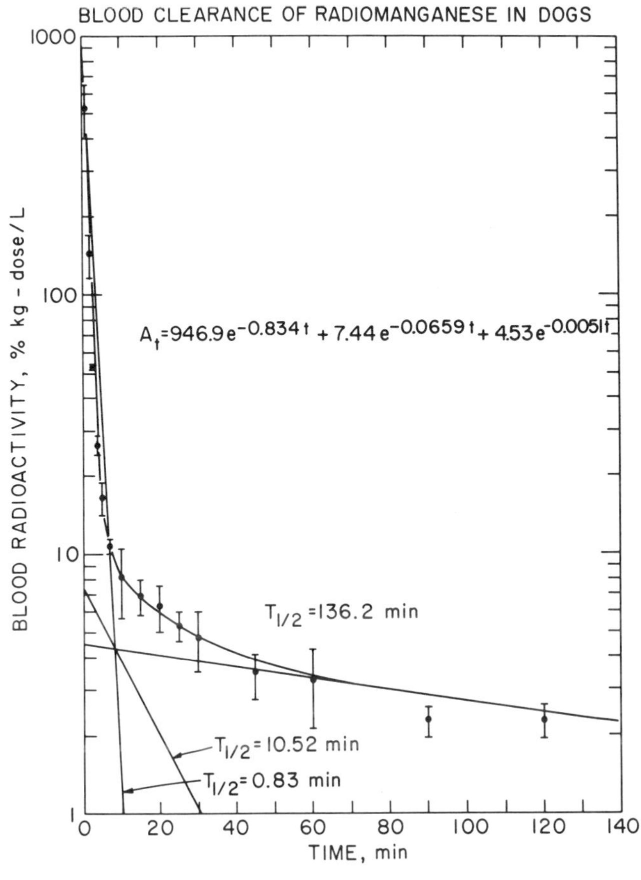

Figure 4. Clearance of $(Mn\text{-}54)Cl_2$ from blood in four dogs. (Reproduced with permission from Ref. 2. Copyright 1979, Radiological Society of America, Inc.)

Xe-122/I-122

A variety of radioisotopes of iodine (I-123, -125, -131) have been shown to be very useful in a wide range of medical applications. However, there remains a gap because of the non-availability of an iodine isotope with a very short half-life for repeat studies in sequence with high photon flux and low dose. Using a short-lived iodine label would thus add these advantages to the long list of existing iodine radiopharmaceuticals. Iodine-122 would appear to fulfill these criteria as well as offering the advantage of the quantitative estimation possible with a positron emitting nuclide. The decay scheme of the Xe-122/I-122 combination is shown in Figure 5.

Method. Presently, the parent xenon-122 is produced in our laboratory as a by-product in the production of xenon-123 for the preparation of high purity iodine-123. The target is a 3.1 g/cm^2 sodium iodide pellet sealed in a 5 cm diameter Inconel ring with 0.025 cm Inconel windows. The target is irradiated in the BLIP with 68-48 MeV protons at a beam current of about 50 μA. Details of the targetry, irradiation, and processing apparatus have been previously reported (7). Multicurie amounts of Xe-123, as well as smaller quantities of other radioxenons (Table II) are produced in a two-hour bombardment. Although the proton energy is not optimum for the I-127(p,6n)Xe-122 reaction, useful quantities of Xe-122 can be made with such a short bombardment. The production yield of Xe-122, measured from the annihilation gammas of I-122, is about 100 mCi at EOB. For a larger quantity of Xe-122, it would probably be necessary to lengthen bombardments and increase the proton energy slightly.

Following the decay period which is required for the production of I-123, the excess xenon activity, including xenon-121, -122, -123, -125, and -127, is transferred to a collection vessel held at liquid nitrogen temperature. After waiting several hours to allow Xe-121 ($t_{1/2}$ = 38.8 minutes) to decay, the remaining xenon is purified by cryogenic pumping through a 2 cm dia. x 5 cm quartz furnace containing titanium sponge (Consolidated Astronautics, Inc., Long Island City, New York) heated to 800°C. Prior to each use, the titanium is thoroughly degassed under vacuum at the same temperature. The xenon isotopes are not affected by the titanium furnace as the noble gases pass through, while traces of other gases are quantitatively removed. This decontamination procedure greatly improves the efficiency of xenon transfer during the I-122 milking process. The xenon is subsequently condensed and isolated in a storage reservoir ready for use with the generator. The reservoir consists of a bellows valve and a stainless steel tube (0.95 cm O.D., 0.80 cm I.D.). The presence of xenon-127 does not affect the radionuclidic quality of I-122

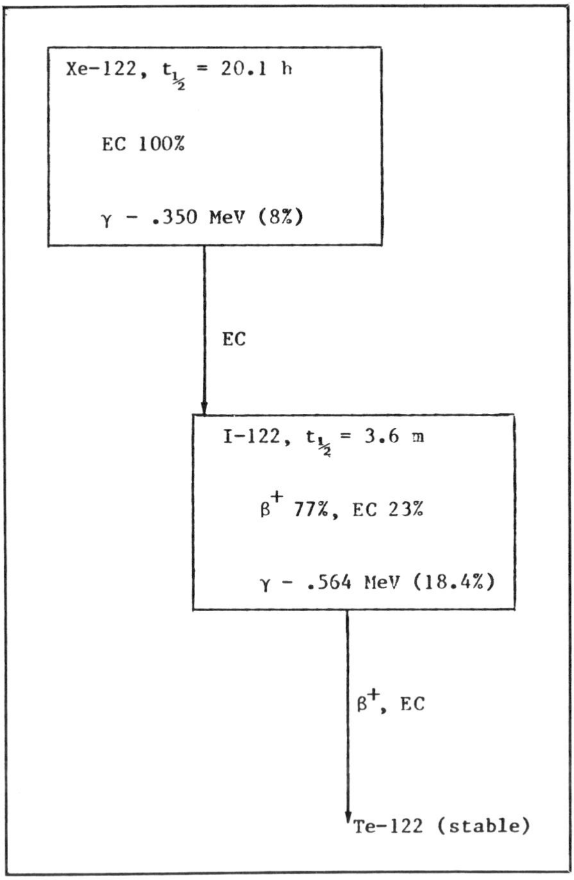

Figure 5. Xe-122/I-122 decay characteristics.

Table II. Radioxenons Produced by 68 MeV Protons in NaI

Nuclear Reaction	Radionuclide	Half-Life	Daughter (Half-life)
(p,n)	Xe-127	36.41 d	I-127 (stable)
(p,3n)	Xe-125	17.0 h	I-125 (60.2 d)
(p,5n)	Xe-123	2.08 h	I-123 (13.0 h)
(p,6n)	Xe-122	20.1 h	I-122 (3.6 m)
(p,7n)	Xe-121	38.8 min	I-121 (2.12 h)

since it decays into stable iodine-127. Iodines from other xenon contaminants such as Xe-123 and Xe-125 are controlled by the short ingrowth period for the iodine-122. For example, starting with equal activity levels of Xe-122, -123 and -125, if the xenon gas remains in the decay vessel for 5, 10 or 15 minutes, the activity of the daughter iodines will be in the ratio 100:0.72:0.006, 100:1.08:0.012, and 100:1.35:0.017 for I-122, 123,and 125 respectively. There would be 29% more I-122 with a 10 minute growth period and 53% more with a 15 minute interval as compared to the 5 minute growth time. Of course, in a practical situation the generator would not be used until the day after production so that the levels of Xe-123, and -125 would be considerably less than assumed in this example.

The generator assembly consists of the above mentioned xenon reservoir and a glass milking vessel (1.30 cm O.D., 1.05 cm I.D.) (Figure 6). The two are connected by means of an L-shaped stainless steel tube (0.64 cm O.D., 0.45 cm I.D.). The top of the milking chamber is a rubber septum held in place by an aluminum seal. For the purpose of transferring the I-122 solution out of the chamber, the vessel is equipped with an inner delivery tube (0.64 cm O.D., 0.12 cm I.D.) which is connected to the outlet side arm (0.64 cm O.D., 0.12 cm I.D.). This tubing points straight down the center with the opening barely touching the conical bottom of the chamber. Attached to the side arm is mounted a toggle valve which is used to isolate the system. The space available in the milking chamber is about 4.5 cm^3. Prior to use, the unit is thoroughly washed with distilled water, methanol, and then vacuum dried.

The milking procedure is as follows: The milking chamber is evacuated to less than 1 μm and then isolated by closing the toggle valve. By maintaining this chamber at liquid nitrogen temperature and opening the bellows valve, Xe-122 is transferred into the chamber and condensed onto the glass wall. At the end of a five- to ten-minute ingrowth period, the liquid nitrogen dewar under the vessel is replaced with a warm water dewar and at the same time the xenon reservoir is cooled with liquid nitrogen. Xenon immediately transfers back to the reservoir while I-122 remains in the dewar. The bellows valve is then closed followed by injecting 2 ml of 1.39% sodium bicarbonate solution through the rubber septum. The toggle valve is subsequently opened to allow the I-122 solution to be drawn into a collection bottle under vacuum via polyethylene tubing. The vacuum also serves to remove any radioxenon remaining in the unfilled space in the bottle. The milking operation can be repeated as desired by replacing the glass vessel with a pretreated spare unit.

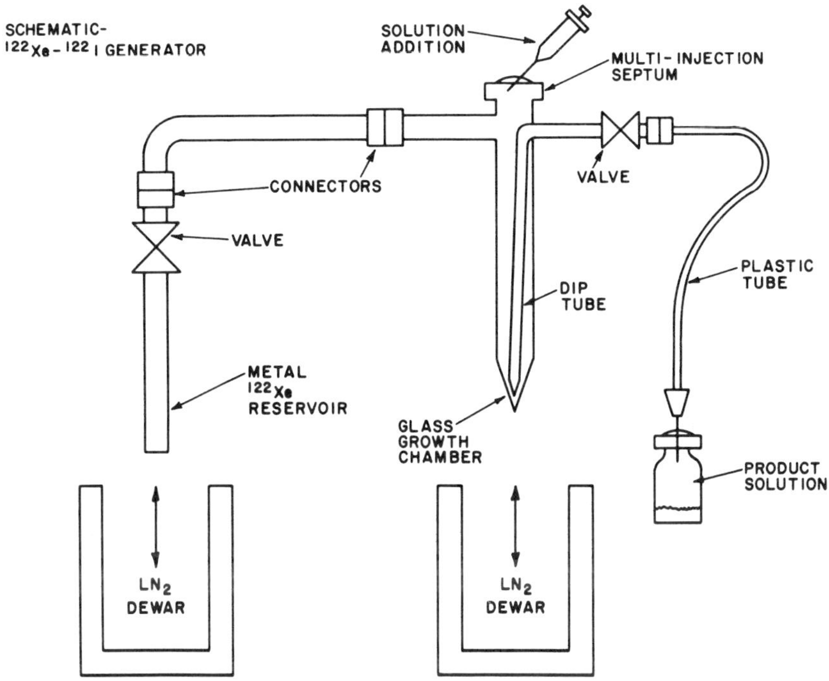

Figure 6. Schematic representation of I-122 generator. (Reproduced with permission from Ref. 7. Copyright 1979, Pergamon Press Ltd.)

The xenon storage reservoir and the ingrowth vessel are kept in two cylindrical lead shields. The entire asembly is constructed on top of a heavy-duty cart. The shields can be partially opened for the mounting and dismounting of the two units. The whole milking operation, including opening and closing the valves, raising and lowering the dewars, and injecting the sodium bicarbonate solution, is performed with the shields closed to provide adequate shielding for the operator. This generator is unique since once constructed it remains at the place of use and is recharged with Xe-122 as needed by attaching a fresh Xe-122 ampoule to the assembly.

The only radionuclidic impurity detected in the I-122 is less than 0.1% radioxenons and other radioiodines, which neither interfere with scintigraphic imaging nor result in a high radiation exposure to the patient. Further improvement of the radioiodine contamination could be attained with an iodine trap between the storage reservoir and the growth chamber. The milking efficiency is about 40%. We consider this generator assembly to be a preliminary version that can be refined considerably. Further details may be obtained from Richards and Ku (8).

Rapid iodinations. To fully exploit the physical advantages offered by I-122, rapid iodination procedures must be developed. These methods must yield high labeling efficiency and unchanged biological behavior of the labeled compound. Initial attempts at rapid iodinations in this laboratory have produced encouraging results (9). Preliminary efforts concentrated on lactoperoxidase catalyzed iodinations and chloramine-T oxidation of iodide. With these procedures it was demonstrated that 85-95% iodination yields with human serum albumin (HSA) in one to three minutes could be achieved upon a proper selection of reaction conditions. Using the lactoperoxidase methods under mild conditions, I-125 HSA was prepared with 88% yield in 1 minute, and 96% after a quick ion-exchange purification. When injected into dogs, 85% of this preparation remained in the blood circulation after 60 minutes. Similarly, a modified chloramine-T procedure gave a 94% yield, and this product had a blood clearance curve in dogs very similar to that obtained using commercial radioiodinated human serum albumin.

Despite the short 3.6-minute half-life, preliminary studies indicate that the biodistribution of I-122 can be followed to determine blood pools of selected organs. The equilibration time for the heart blood pool is less than two minutes; for the lung blood pool, this time is even shorter. Thus, two to three half-lives is adequate to investigate these pools by using I-122 labeled albumin. The extension of rapid iodination procedures to labeling compounds known to have specific physiological function in other organs would significantly enhance the usefulness of iodine-122.

Te-118/Sb-118

At this time our interest in this potential generator system is motivated primarily by the attractive radionuclidic properties summarized in Figure 7. Tellurium-118 decays 100% by electron capture with no gamma emissions. The 3.5 minute Sb-118 daughter has very modest gamma emissions; the most significant gamma photon is only 2.5% abundant (1.230 MeV). Additionally, Te-118 represents a bonus since it can be produced in an antimony target simultaneously with tin-117m. The BLIP production of Sn-117m in a carrier-free form is an ongoing project to study the in-vivo behavior of tin compounds (10).

The relevant nuclear reaction for tellurium is primarily Sb-121(p,4n)Te-118 with some contribution from the (p,6n) reaction on Sb-123 (42.7% abundance). The nuclear excitation functions for these reactions have not been measured. A series of stacked foil irradiations is planned to determine thin target cross sections. This will allow selection of optimal bombardment parameters for thick target irradiation at the BLIP. A calculated excitation function for the (p,4n) reaction is shown in Figure 8. This calculation is based on the interpolation method of Munzel et al. (11) and should allow prediction of thick target yields to within a factor of 2 or 3.

The no carrier added chemical separation of both tellurium and tin from a large antimony target is difficult. Dissolving the massive target itself is something of a problem as aqua regia and hot concentrated sulfuric acid work only slowly and can lead to insoluble precipitates without careful control of solution volume and temperature. Instead, concentrated HCl with liquid bromine has been used. This solution is then diluted with water to about 2*N* HCl. Antimony oxychloride precipitates, beginning at 4*N* HCl. Approximately 85% of the antimony radioactivity, most of the tellurium and none of the tin are to be found in the precipitate. After filtering, the filtrate is added to an anion exchange column for further purification of the tin-117m. The precipitate is redissolved in concentrated HCl and the solution is adjusted to about 5*N* HCl. Selenium carrier is added and the solution is then saturated with SO_2 to precipitate elemental selenium (carries Te radioactivity). After filtration the selenium is dissolved in concentrated HNO_3 and concentrated HBr is added. This solution is evaporated by heating to remove the selenium as $SeBr_4$. The remaining tellurium can be dissolved in a small volume of oxidizing acid. This procedure, although successful is still being refined. The investigation of a suitable generator column is now being initiated.

A preliminary non-optimal irradiation (1 hr) of a 36 g antimony target was attempted at an incident energy of 58 MeV. The measured EOB yield of Te-118 was 9.5 μCi/g-μAh. Thus, Curie quantities could easily be produced with a several day bombardment at 50 μA. Preliminary analyses of the other tellurium radioactivities produced are summarized in Table III.

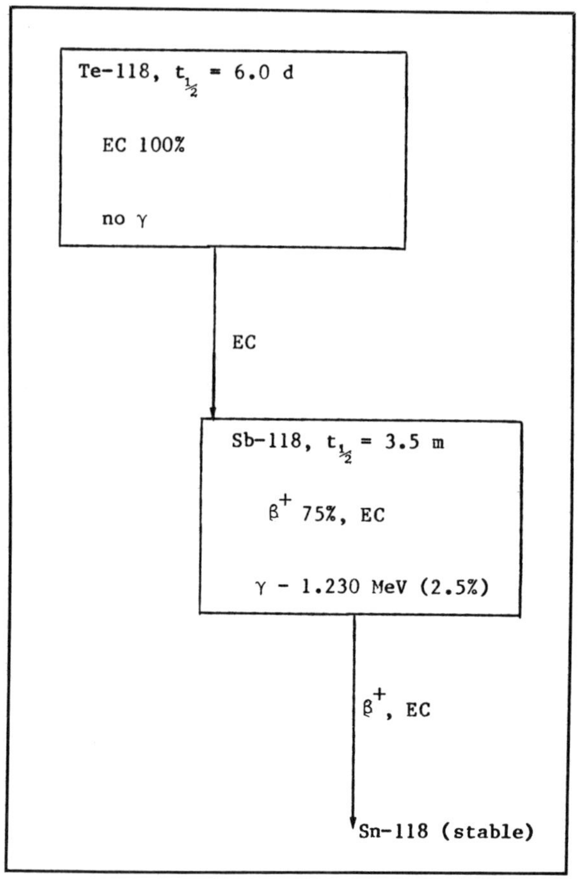

Figure 7. Te-118/Sb-118 decay characteristics.

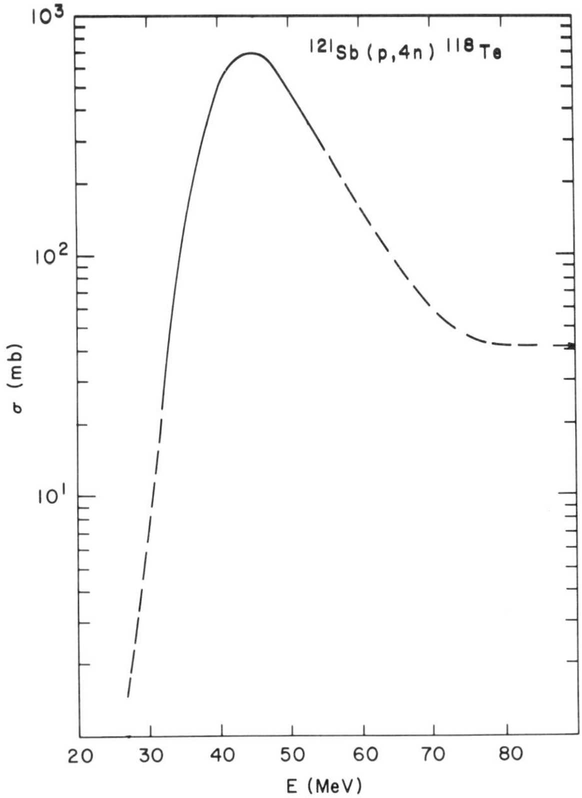

Figure 8. Calculated excitation function of Sb-121(p,4n)Te-118 reaction.

Table III. Production Rate of Te Nuclides in Sb at 58 MeV (μCi/g-μAh)

Te-118	Te-119	Te-121	Te-121m	Te-123
9.5	12.0	0.54	0.096	0.11

Under different, optimized reaction conditions these quantities will change. In a generator system Te-123m represents no problem since it decays to stable Te-123 which would remain on the column. Also, both Te-121m and Te-121 decay to stable Sb-121. However, Te-119 leads to Sb-119 which has a half-life of 38 hours. The amount of Sb-119 eluted with the Sb-118 can be minimized by taking advantage of their large difference in half-life. That is, in operation a pre-elution should be performed to clean the column of antimony. After 20 minutes, Sb-118 has regained equilibrium with minimal ingrowth of Sb-119. In this manner the Sb-119 can be controlled to less than 0.7% of the desired antimony-118.

At this early stage the primary application of this generator system appears to be for angiography. The 3.5 minute half-life is more convenient to handle for bolus injection than 30 second gold-195m. Due to finite circulation time, the slower decay should presumably allow better imaging of the left ventricle. There might also be sufficient time to perform some chemistry on the antimony - perhaps to prepare colloids with potential utilization for studying liver regional blood flow and clearance.

Conclusion

Three new positron emitting generator systems have been described. The practical availability of these radionuclides could significantly broaden the potential applications of positron emission tomography. The next few years should see human clinical trials undertaken to fully evaluate their utility for nuclear medicine.

Acknowledgment

We would like to acknowledge the support of this work by the U.S. Department of Energy under Contract #DE-AC02-76CH00016.

Literature Cited

1. Chauncey, D.M.; Schelbert, H.R.; Halpern, S.E.; Delano, F.; McKegney, M.L.; Ashburn, W.L.; Hagan, P.L. J. Nucl. Med. 1977, 18, 933-936.
2. Atkins, H.L.; Som, P.; Fairchild, R.G.; Hui, J.; Schachner, E.; Goldman, A.; Ku, T.H. Radiol. 1979, 133, 769-774.
3. Atcher, R.W.; Friedman, A.M.; Huizenga, J.R.; Rayudu, G.V.S.; Silverstein, E.A.; Turner, D.A. J.Nucl. Med. 1978, 19, 689.
4. Richards, P.; Lebowitz, E.; Stang, L.G. Radiopharmaceuticals and Labeled Compounds IAEA, Vienna, Vol 1, 1973, 325-341.

5. Ku, T.H.; Richards, P.; Stang, L.G.; Prach, T. Radiol. 1979, 132, 475-477.
6. Hui, J.; Atkins, H.L.; Som, P.; Ku, T.H.; Fairchild, R.G.; Giwa, L.O.; Richards, P. J. Nucl. Med. 1979, 20, 648.
7. Richards, P.; Prach, T.; Srivastava, S.C.; Meinken, G.E. J. Radioanal. Chem. 1981, 65, 47-50.
8. Richards, P.; Ku, T.H. Int. J. Appl. Rad. Isot. 1979, 30, 250-254.
9. Srivastava, S.C., personal communication.
10. Srivastava, S.C.; Richards, P.; Meinken, G.E.; Som, P.; Knapp, Jr., F.F.; Butler, T.A. Proc. 3rd World Cong. Nucl. Med. Biol. 1982, p. 1635-1638.
11. Munzel, H.; Lange, J.; Keller, J.A. "Q-values and excitation functions of nuclear reactions" Landolt-Bornstein New Series, I 15 Part C.

RECEIVED August 19, 1983

7

An Automated Microprocessor-Controlled Rb-82 Generator for Positron Emission Tomography Studies

Y. YANO, T. F. BUDINGER, J. L. CAHOON, and R. H. HUESMAN

Donner Laboratory and Lawrence Berkeley Laboratory, University of California, Berkeley, CA 94720

Radioisotope generators provide a desirable alternative to cyclotrons for the production of short lived positron emitters. A fully automated microprocessor controlled generator system for obtaining 76 sec rubidium-82 is described in detail. Column adsorbants, specifications and eluent solutions are discussed in determining generator performance for yield, breakthrough, and stability for long term use. Some examples of clinical applications in positron emission tomography are presented.

Ultra short lived radionuclides, with a half-life of a few seconds to a few minutes are readily available from long-lived parent radionuclides adsorbed to an organic or inorganic ion exchange support matrix (1-3). These radionuclide generator systems are an inexpensive alternative to an on-site cyclotron, especially for positron emitters used for positron emission tomography (PET). In PET studies it is an advantage to have very short half life positron emitters which permit the administration of 10-20 mCi of radioactivity for good statistical sampling in the reconstructed cross-sectional image while minimizing the radiation dose to the patient. An added benefit of the short half life is the rapid decay of background activity within 5-10 minutes. Repeat studies can then be performed on the same subject to obtain additional information under different physiological conditions. Some generators for positron emitters are listed in Table I. Generator produced Ga-68 is of considerable interest because of its potential for imaging thrombi formation with labeled platelets and for imaging atheroma with bifunctinal chelate labeled lipoproteins (4,5). Bifunctional chelates are also applicable to labeling monoclonal antibodies. Other positron emitters from generators, which have been studied, are Ba-128/Cs-128 (6), Fe-52/Mn-52m (7,8), and Zn-62/Cu-62 (9). The Xe-122/I-122 generator can be useful in labeling amphetamine analogs with I-122 to measure brain

0097-6156/84/0241-0097$07.50/0
© 1984 American Chemical Society

Table I. Generators for Positron Emitters

Parent	Half-life	Decay Mode(%)	Daughter	Half-life	Decay Mode(%)	Gamma MeV(%)
Fe-52	8.3 h	β^+(56),EC(44)	Mn-52 m	21.1 m	β^+(98),EC(2)	1.43(100)
Zn-62	9.1 h	β^+(18),EC(82)	Cu-62	9.8 m	β^+(100)	0.59(22)
Ge-68	275 d	EC(100)	Ga-68	68 m	β^+(88),EC(12)	1.08(3.5)
Sr-82	25 d	EC(100)	Rb-82	76 s	β^+(96),EC(4)	0.73(9)
Te-118	6.0 d	EC(100)	Sb-118	3.5 m	β^+(75),EC(22)	1.23(3)
Xe-122	20.1 h	EC(100)	I-122	3.5 m	β^+(100)	0.56(14)
Ba-128	2.43 d	EC(100)	Cs-128	3.8 m	β^+(51),EC(49)	0.44(27)

blood flow by PET (10,11). This chapter will discuss experience with the strontium-82/rubidium-82 generator and its operation in the automated mode for PET studies.

Experimental Studies

Rubidium-82 Generator Development. The radionuclidic properties of the 76 sec Rb-82 and the 25 day Sr-82 parent are shown in the decay scheme, Figure 1. Strontium-82 decays 100% by electron capture (E.C.) to the 1.25 min Rb-82, which decays 96% by β^+ emission and 4% by E.C. to the ground state of Kr-82. The 511 keV annihilation photons are accompanied by a 777 keV gamma emission in 13% abundance. The β^+_{max} energy is 3.35 MeV.

The first Rb-82 generator was developed in 1968 with a weakly acidic cation exchange resin, Bio Rex 70, and ammonium acetate as the eluent solution (12). The development of the Rb-82 generator over a period of 14 years is outlined in Table II. Other Rb-82 generator systems were developed which used the chelating ion exchange resin, Chelex 100, and an NH_4OH-NH_4Cl eluent (13), alumina the inorganic ion exchanger (14,15) and zirconium oxide (16) using saline as the eluent solution. Recent Rb-82 generators have used a combination of alumina and Chelex 100 in tandem columns (17,18) and a SnO_2 column (19,20). Normal saline or 1.8% NaCl solutions were used as the eluent solution. The alumina column was used in an automated microprocessor controlled system (21).

The Rb-82 generator permits serial studies in the same patient as often as every 10 minutes with 20-60 mCi of Rb-82 for rapid bolus intravenous infusion. Inherent in the administration of high levels of Rb-82 activity is the need for precise flow control from an automated system to deliver the desired amount of radioactivity. The development of the alumina column parameters and the elution protocol as well as the automated microprocessor system controller are presented here. Some of the details of this system have been discussed in earlier publications (15,21). Generator produced Rb-82 is used as a diffusible flow tracer in myocardial perfusion studies and as a nondiffusible tracer in brain studies to assess blood brain barrier permeability changes in patients with brain tumors or Alzheimer's type dementia.

Production of Sr-82. An important consideration in the development of radioisotope generators is the availability, cost, and radionuclidic purity of the long-lived parent. In the case of Sr-82, the 25 day radionuclide is needed in 100-200 mCi amounts in order to provide adequate elution yields of Rb-82 from one loading of Sr-82 every three months. Initially the Sr-82 for the generator was produced at the Lawrence Berkeley Laboratory (LBL) 88-inch cyclotron by the Rb-85 (p,4n) Sr-82 nuclear reaction (12). However, because of the long irradiation time required to produce

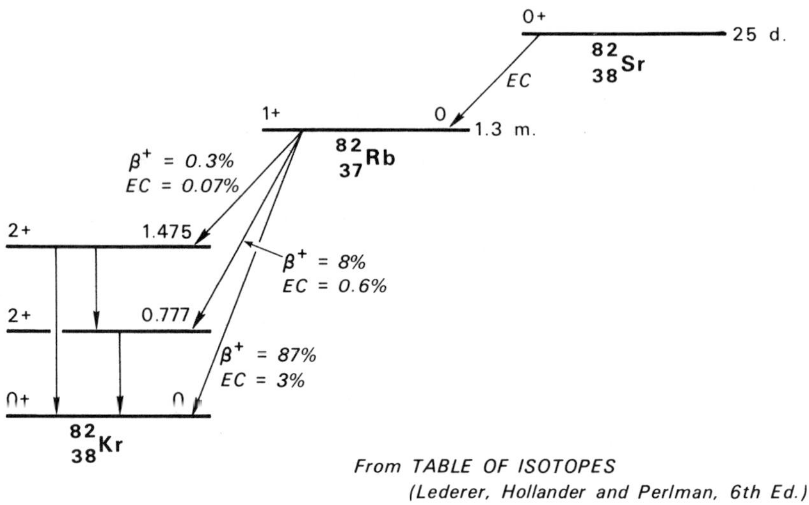

Figure 1. Sr-82/Rb-82 decay scheme.

Table II. Rubidium-82 Generators

Column	Eluent	Rb-82 Yield (%)	Sr-82/85 Breakthrough/ml	Reference
Bio-Rex 70	NH_4Ac	72	10^{-5}	Yano 1968
Chelex 100	NH_4Cl	90	10^{-7}	Grant 1975
Bio-Rex 70	NaCl	72	10^{-7}	Yano 1979
Al_2O_3	NaCl	76	10^{-7}	Yano 1979
ZrO_2	NaCl	60-70	10^{-8}	Kulprathipanja 1979
Al_2O_3 + Chelex 100	NaCl	14-66	10^{-9}	Horlock 1981
Al_2O_3	NaCl	80-90	10^{-8}	Yano 1981
SnO2	NaCl	70	10^{-9}	Neirinckx 1981
Al_2O_3 + Chelex 100	NaCl	40	10^{-9}	Vallabhajousla 1981

mCi amounts of Sr-82, this method was too costly for routine production of large quantities of Sr-82. Fortunately, the high to medium energy protons from the linear accelerators at the Los Alamos National Laboratory and the Brookhaven National Laboratory (BNL) are available to produce Sr-82 and other useful radionuclides in high yields.

The Sr-82 used in these studies was produced by spallation of a molybdenum target with 800 MeV protons at the Los Alamos Meson Physics Facility (LAMPF) and radiochemically separated by the Nuclear Chemistry Group at Los Alamos Scientific Laboratory (LASL) (22). The major radionuclidic contaminant in the Sr-82 is Sr-85 which is present in at least 1:1 ratio relative to Sr-82. The actual ratio depends upon the length of time after the production of radioactive strontium. Because of the 65 day half life of Sr-85 and the 25 day half life of Sr-82, the Sr-85:Sr-82 ratio increases with time. Other radionuclides found by the Hammersmith group in the processed Sr-82/85 shipment were Sr-89 (1%), Sr-90 (0.01%), Co-58 (1%) and Rb-84 (1%) from (17).

Alumina Column Yields and Breakthrough. Previous experience with the basic alumina column for the Rb-82 generator led to the design of the present column (15). The yield of Rb-82 in the column eluent is dependent on the Al_2O_3 bed volume, concentration of saline eluent, and flow-rate. These parameters also affect the breakthrough of Sr. Figures 2a and 2b show the effect of these factors for an alumina column of 0.25 to 1.00 ml, using saline solutions 1.25 to 2.00% in NaCl (15). For the 2% NaCl eluent there was a factor of 100 less breakthrough for a 25% increase in column volume from 0.75 to 1.00 ml. In the case of 1.25% NaCl eluent a 25% increase in column volume resulted in a tenfold decrease in breakthrough. The yield of Rb-82 from a 1 ml bed volume was increased by about 10% for 1.75-2.00% NaCl concentration compared to the 1.25-1.50% NaCl. The breakthrough of Al_2O_3 was 5 μg/ml of 2.0% NaCl of pH 8-9. This value is one-half the allowable breakthrough for Al_2O_3 for a Tc-99m generator of 10 μg/ml as set by the national regulatory agency. Because of the large amounts of radioactivity (200 mCi Sr-82 and 300-400 mCi of Sr-85) in the automated generators, a larger volume of Al_2O_3 was used is these studies to minimize breakthrough over long term use of the generator.

A stainless steel (ss) tube 3/8" o.d. with 1/16" wall thickness and 10 cm long (3.2 ml) is fitted with ss screens and Millipore prefilters at the top and bottom of the stainless steel (ss) tube which is connected by 3/8" to 1/8" Swagelok reducers to 1/8" o.d. ss tubing. All of the column components are autoclaved and assembled. The top connector and screen are removed and the column is filled with 100-200 mesh Bio-Rad basic alumina in a water slurry at pH 8-9. The alumina column is clamped between two rectangular lead plates that have been machined to fit around the ss column and placed inside of a solid lead cylinder 5 inches in

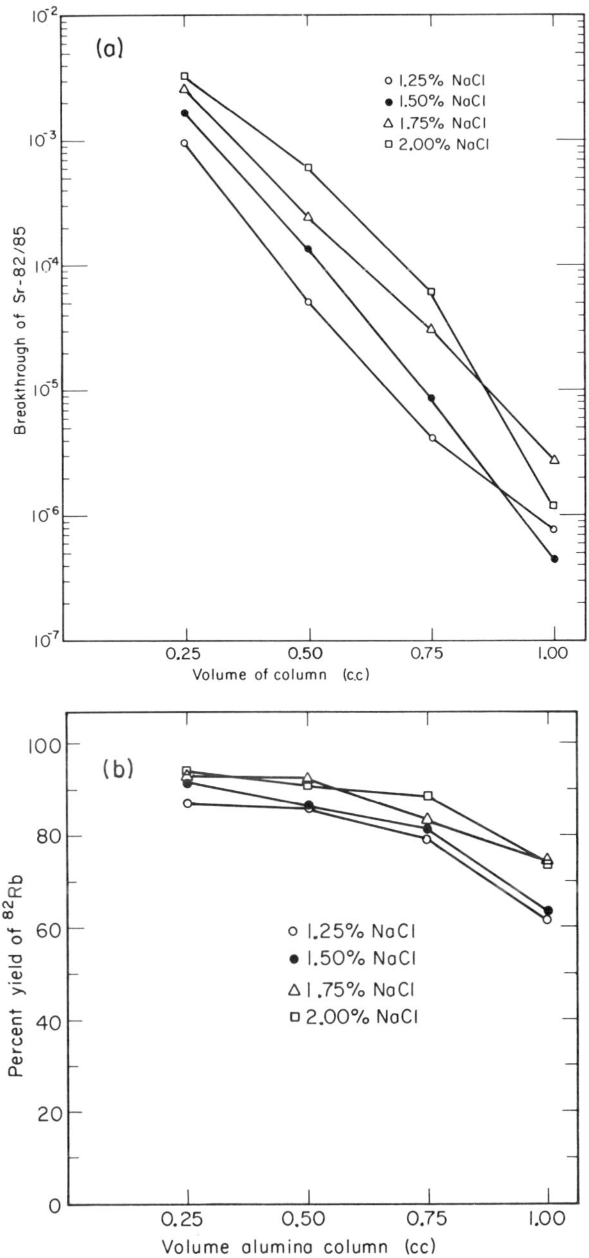

Figure 2. Effects of Al_2O_3 column volumes and NaCl concentration in Rb-82 generator elutions. (Reproduced with permission from Ref. 15. Copyright 1979, J. Nucl. Med.)

diameter which has been slotted to accept the rectangular plate column shield. The shield and column are placed in a lucite enclosure behind the "hot cell" for remote pumping and loading of the Sr-82/85 as shown in Figure 3.

Loading Sr-82/85. The Sr-82/85 is shipped in a few ml of dilute HCl from LASL. The shipping shield is opened remotely and the contents of the vial are transferred to a flask. The Sr-82/85 solution is diluted with about 100 ml sterile pyrogen-free H_2O to maintain a low salt concentration and the pH is adjusted to 8-9 with dilute base. A remotely operated pumping system pumps the Sr-82/85 solution through the alumina column at a flow rate of about 1-2 ml/min. After the Sr-82/85 has been placed on the column, the flask and pumping syringe are washed two times with about 40 ml of pH 8-9 sterile water. Usually the column is left undisturbed overnight to allow the Sr-82/85 to become more firmly fixed to the alumina matrix. The column is then purged with 500 ml of 2% saline at pH 8-9 at a moderate flow rate of about 0.5 ml/sec. Quick-connects allow the column and shielding to be easily freed from the pump and connecting lines.

Construction and Operation of the Rb-82 Generator. The Sr-82/85 column and shield are then transported to the PET imaging site and the Sr-82/85 shield is lifted into a secondary lead cyclinder with 3 inch wall thickness. Quick connects are used to connect the column to the lines from the automated and microprocessor controlled pumping unit as shown in Figure 4a. An open loop (Slo-Syn) stepping motor is used to provide adequate torque and a wide dynamic speed range. A timing belt connects the stepping motor to a recirculating ball-nut and screw that moves the stainless steel piston inside of the specially machined Lexan barrel. A Bellofram rolling diaphram around the piston provides a low friction seal against airborne contamination and prevents the saline eluent solution from contacting the stainless steel piston. The motor controller is a 6800 Motorola microprocessor with 4K memory, a crystal clock, a programmable timing module, two RS-232 serial ports, and an 8-bit analog to digital converter. The controller converts input from the operator into a precise number of pulses for the stepping motor. The micro processor minimizes operator error by simplifying the controls and doing the calculations, counting, and timing. The schematic of the controller is shown in Figure 4-b.

The front panel of the controller has two four-digit thumbwheel switches and two lighted pushbutton switches. The thumbwheels determine flow rate (ml/min) and volume to be delivered (ml). One pushbutton switch initiates the pump-refill operation. The other starts the injection, or stops an injection in progress. After power-up or reset, the microprocessor initializes itself and sets up the timing module and serial ports. It then jumps into a looping program that scans the two pushbutton switches and the

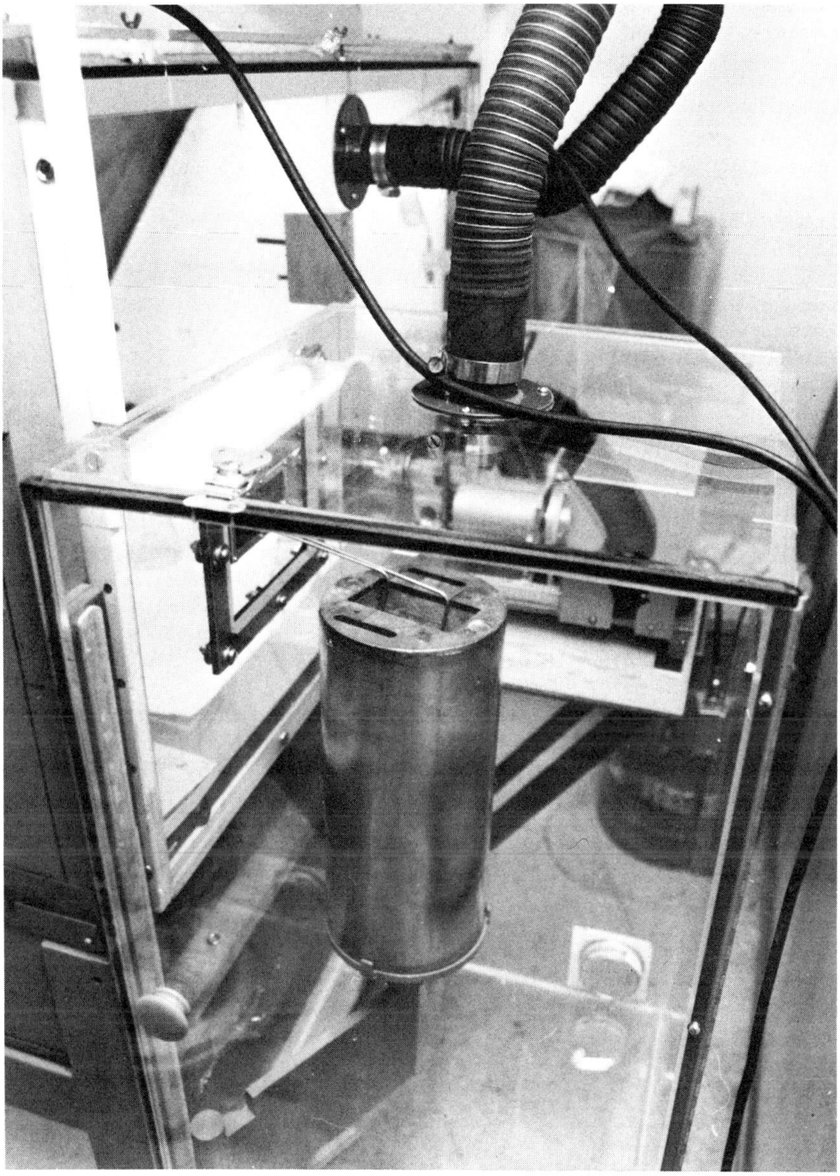

Figure 3. Alumina column in primary lead shielding in position for loading with Sr-82.

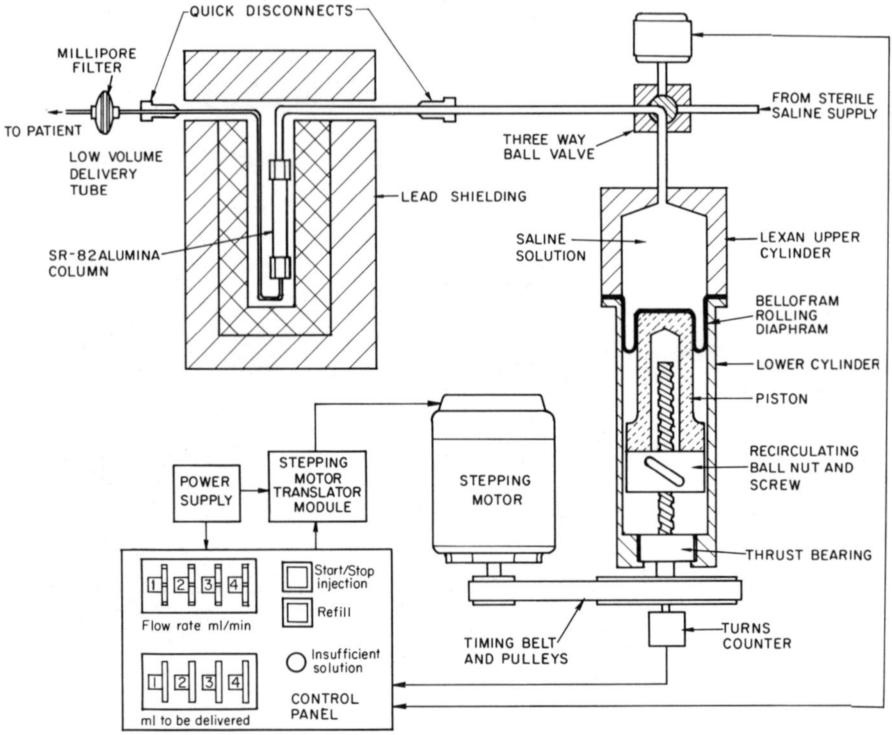

Figure 4a. Automated Rb-82 generator with microprocessor control. (Reproduced with permission from Ref. 21. Copyright 1981, J. Nucl. Med.)

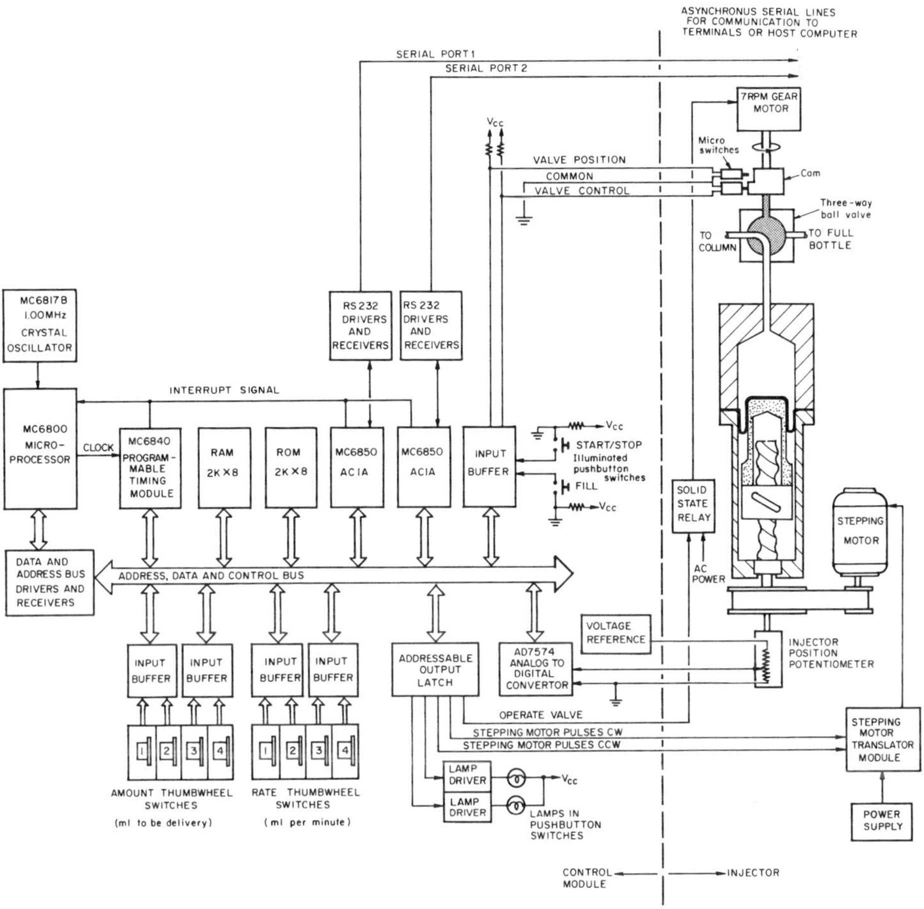

Figure 4b. Schematic of microprocessor controller.

thumbwheel switch specifying volume. The system thus monitors changes in switch settings, scanning at greater than 1000 times per second. When a change is detected, the new setting is stored and the program enters a service routine for that particular switch. The first part of each routine is a delay that guarantees that the new setting is stable for at least 50 msec.

Another part of the loop program ascertains how much solution is left in the pump. A voltage picked off a ten-turn potentiometer, which is coupled to the piston-drive screw with a timing belt, is fed to the analog-to-digital converter and is compared with the previously stored reading from the thumbwheel switch. If the operator has requested a greater volume of solution than present in the pump, the program sets up a circuit in the programmable timing module that causes the insufficient lamp to flash twice a second. An injection cannot be started in this state; the operator must either refill the pump from the solution reservoir or change the amount to be delivered. The outlet from the pump is connected to a motor-driven three-way valve by 1/8" ss tubing and Swagelok fittings. The three-way valve allows connection to either the saline fill bottle when the controller is in the refill position or to the Sr-82/Rb-82 alumina column when the controller is in the elution position.

The filling sequence is started when the loop program has determined that the fill pushbutton has been actuated. The fill service routine turns on the refill pushbutton light, turns on the valve motor and waits for the correct valve position, then sends 100-sec pulses to the stepping motor in the reverse direction until the pump reservoir is filled; it then turns on the valve motor again, waits for correct position, turns off the refill light, and reenters the loop program. The last part of the loop program determines whether the start/stop pushbutton has been activated. If it has, the service routine reads the flow-rate thumbwheel switch and computes the period T during which pulses are sent to the stepping motor, as defined by equation (1), F is flow rate in ml/min and C, a systems constant, is calculated to be 257 pulses to deliver 1 ml of eluent. The quantity of injected solution Q ml (2) is determined by the number of pulses N sent to the stepping motor.

$$T(\text{msec}) = \frac{6 \times 10^4}{FC} \qquad (1)$$

$$Q = \frac{N}{C} \qquad (2)$$

This system will perform both bolus and constant infusion studies with the microprocessor controller. In addition, variable or exponential infusion studies can be performed by using programs residing in a host computer to calculate constants which are sent to the controller through the serial port.

Elution and Breakthrough Characteristics of the Generator. The fractional elution yield and cumulative yield of Rb-82 are shown in Figure 5a,b for 2% saline bolus elutions at a flow rate of 1 ml/sec. Nine 3 ml fractions were collected over 27 sec. Each value is the mean of 3 determinations. Fractions 3-5 contain 70% of the Rb-82 available from the Sr-82 on the alumina column. The total elution yield is about 95% in nine fractions.

In some studies it is desirable to do constant infusion to achieve a steady state or equilibrium condition which is a function of input, extraction rate, tissue washout, and radioactive decay (23). Figure 6 shows the yield of Rb-82 at various elution rates to a steady-state condition. At the faster flow rate of 5.33 ml/min, there is 24% yield of Rb-82 and at the slower flow rate of 2.15 ml/min there is about 1% yield of Rb-82. The lower yield at the slower flow rate is mostly accounted for in decay during transit through the line to the patient.

The advantage of an automated precision flow controlled generator is seen in Figure 7, which shows the relationship between decay of the Sr-82 on the column and the elution time required to deliver a desired radioactive dose of Rb-82 for bolus infusion studies at a flow rate of 1 ml/sec. The elution time in sec is selected and an equivalent volume is set on the thumbwheel switches for volume desired. Normally when the conditions of delivery line volume and column characteristics are unchanged, pre-set values determined from the chart will deliver 95 $\pm$ 5% of the desired radioactive dose. The actual radioactive dose delivered is checked in three preelutions before the beginning of each day of patient studies. The history of a typical column packed with alumina and loaded 3 separate times with Sr-82/85 is shown in Table III. The generator column was used for a period of nine months or an average life of 3 months for each Sr-82 loading. The average breakthrough of Sr-82/85 for each bolus elution was about 10^{-7} for columns 10a and 10b. These columns contained about 600 mCi of Sr-82/85 at maximum activity. Thus, the breakthrough was in the 60 nCi range.

Column 10c contained an unusually large amount of Sr-85 activity of about 2 Ci. To compensate for this heavy loading, a small trapping column of 1.5 ml of alumina was placed down-stream from the main column and the breakthrough was maintained in the 30-40 nCi range. Because of the increased total volume from the addition of the second alumina column, the elution yield of Rb-82 decreased from 78% to 61% in column 10c.

Selected samples of Rb-82 elutions were analyzed for radionuclidic breakthrough by Ge/Li analysis. These results are shown in Table IV. The smaller sample numbers indicate samples taken relatively soon after loading the column with Sr when the breakthroughs are higher. As more elutions were done after the column loading, the breakthroughs of Sr-82/85 and other contaminating radionuclides decreased. Samples 75 and 76 reflect the breakthroughs from column 10c in Table III where the activity of Sr-82

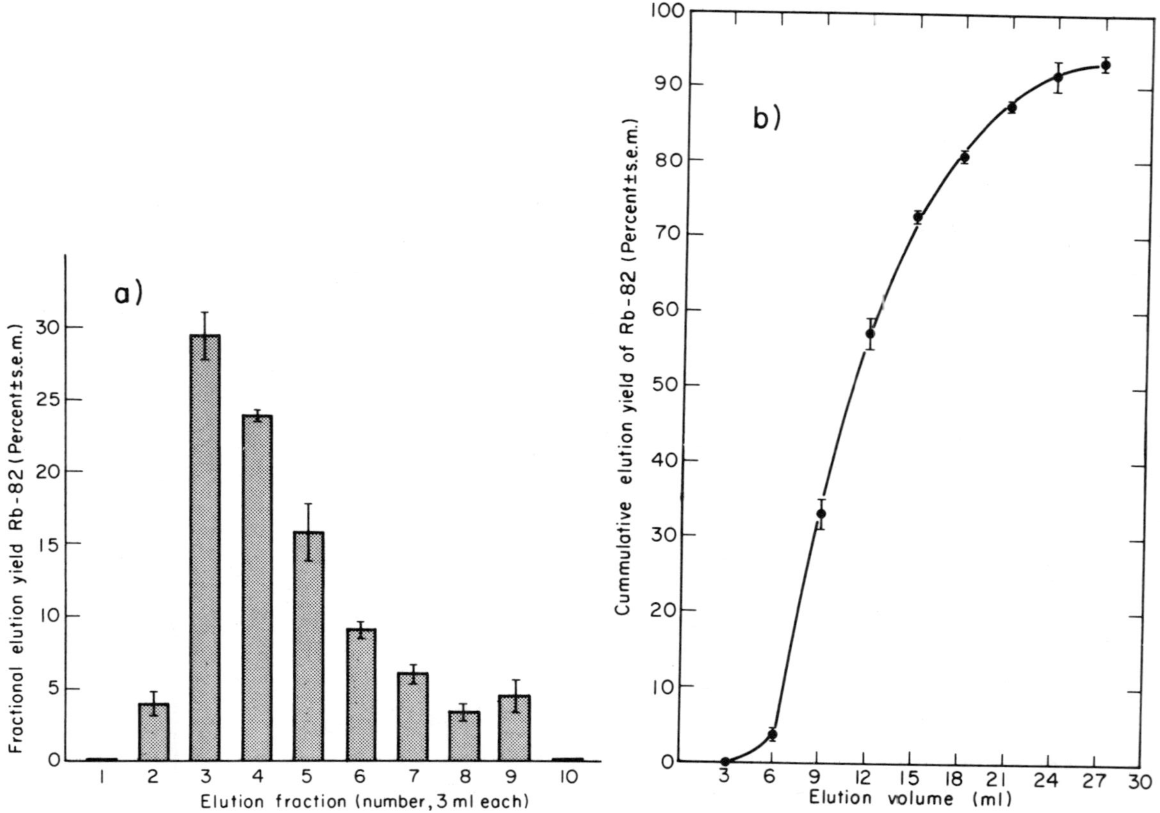

Figure 5. Fractional elution yield of Rb-82 from an alumina column at a flow rate of 1 mL/s and accumulative yield for nine 3-mL fractions, mean of 3 determinations. (Reproduced with permission from Ref. 21. Copyright 1981, J. Nucl. Med.)

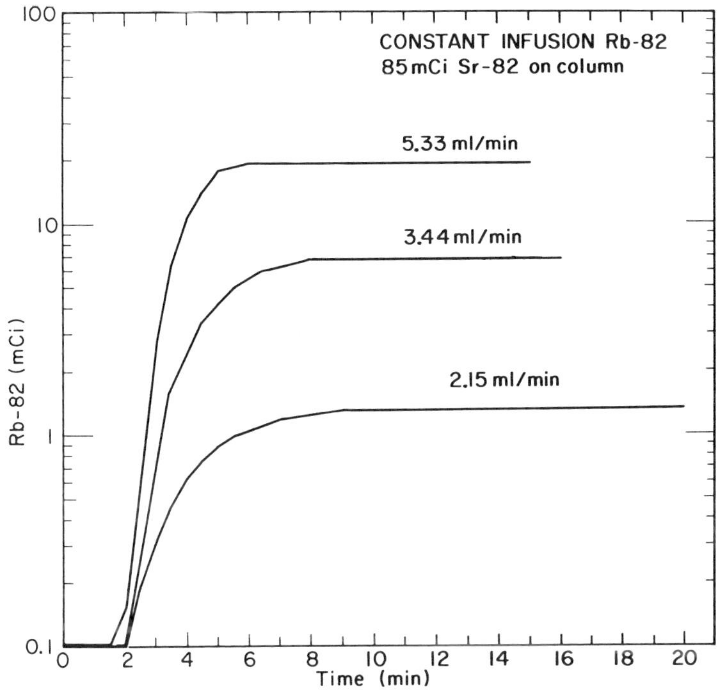

Figure 6. Rb-82 elution yield at steady-state conditions for various flow rates. (Reproduced with permission from Ref. 21. Copyright 1981, J. Nucl. Med.)

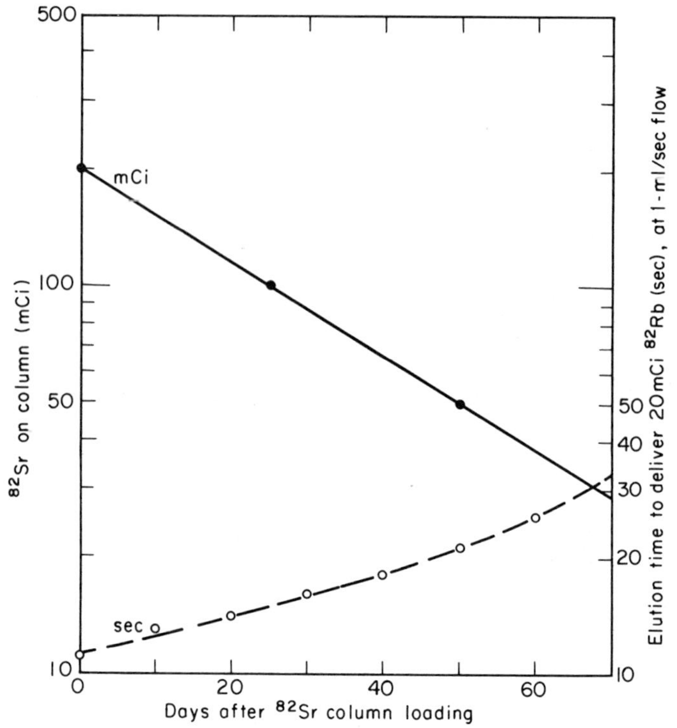

Figure 7. Elution time in s to deliver 20 mCi of Rb-82 for bolus infusion studies at a flow rate of 1 mL/s. (Reproduced with permission from Ref. 21. Copyright 1981, J. Nucl. Med.)

Table III. History of One Alumina Column and Three ^{82}Sr Loadings

Column	Date		Sr Loading (mCi)		Rb-82	Sr Breakthrough
	Start	End	Sr-82	Sr-85	Yield(%)	(range)
10-a	8-26-81	11-20-81	197.5	439	79	$5x4x10^{-8}-1.9x10^{-6}$
10-b	11-13-81	1-18-82	132	460	78	$2.7x10^{-8}-1.7x10^{-6}$
*10-c	1-28-82	6-3-82	175	2,008	61	$5.7x10^{-9}-1.9x10^{-7}$

* Trapping column added

Table IV. Radionuclides in Rb-82 Eluates (nCi/20 ml Elution)

Date	Sample	V-48	Cr-51	Mn-54	Co-57	Co-58	Sr-82/ Rb-82	Rb-83	Sr-85
04/24/81	16	0.30	77.0	0.20		0.04	0.40	44.00	1.20
09/24/81	66		0.90	0.01	0.01	0.01	0.45	0.04	0.90
02/26/82	63			0.05	0.08	0.08	1.30	0.20	22.70
03/01/82	75			0.08	0.08	0.08	1.70	0.95	34.30
03/02/82	76			0.07	0.09	0.14	2.10	0.49	34.10
10/25/82	8	0.01	1.0	0.10			5.5	22	13.6

and Sr-85 is 2 Ci and the breakthrough of Sr-82 and Sr-85 is 36 nCi.

Radiation Dosimetry. The radiation dose to the skeleton of a 70 kg man from 1 μCi of Sr-82/Rb-82 and Sr-85 is reported to be 71 and 7.6 mrads, respectively (17). The estimated radiation dose from 10 mCi of Rb-82 is 700 mrads to kidneys, 140 mrads to heart and 90 mrads to lungs (24). These radiation dose estimations are on the high side and in later calculations have been found to be lower by accounting for decay in vivo in transit to the specific tissues.

Clinical Studies

Heart Studies. Patients are placed in position on the Donner 280 crystal positron tomograph which is a single slice PET system with bismuth germanate (BGO) detectors (25,26). Transmission images are taken with a Ge-68 hoop source and the data are used to correct for attenuation. The patient is connected to the outflow line from the Rb-82 generator by an intravenous catheter and three-way valve. The required time in secs translated into ml required for a 20 mCi dose of Rb-82 is set on the thumbwheel switches of the microprocessor controller. The elution button is pressed in synchrony with the start of data accumulation by the computer of the PET system. For studies of myocardial blood perfusion, gated studies are performed by synchronizing to the R-wave of the electrocardiagram. Data are collected on the selected portion of the cardiac cycle. This is normally triggered on the R-wave to +70 sec. Gated studies sharpen the image by reducing blurring from the movement of the heart and permit the accumulation of input function data from the ventricular blood pool.

Rubidium-82 myocardial perfusion images are used to study patients with myocardial ischemia or infarction. An example of this study is shown in Figure 8. Three patients with known myocardial infarction were imaged with Rb-82. Twenty millicuries of Rb-82 were administered in a 20 ml bolus in 20 sec. Data accumulated from 0-90 seconds post infusion show the blood pool as the radioactivity enters the right side of the heart, flows out to the lungs, and returns to the left side of the heart. Data accumulated from 90-300 seconds reflect uptake of Rb-82 in the myocardium as distributed by blood flow. These results by a non-invasive procedure correlated with the results of catheterized contrast x-ray studies (27,28).

Figure 9 shows the results of two coronary bypass patients studied with Rb-82 and PET. The uptake of Rb-82 is shown in three 1 cm sections of the myocardium. Each section was imaged with a single bolus infusion of 20 mCi Rb-82. Patient A had blood perfusion defects in the mid and lower sections of the myocardium.

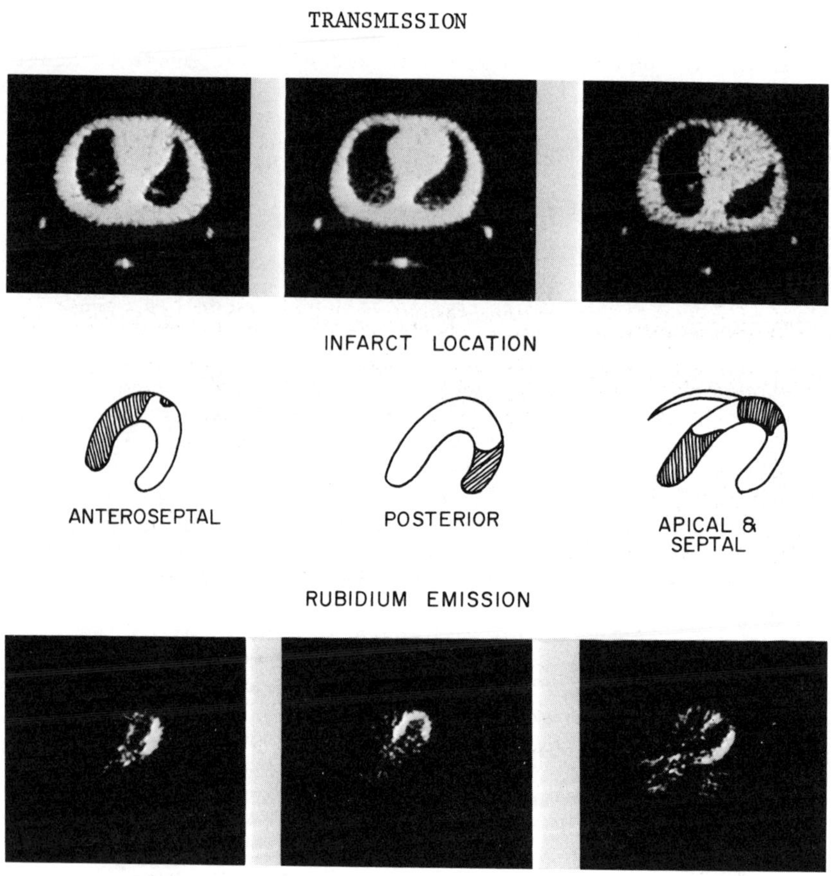

Figure 8. Myocardial perfusion studies with Rb-82 indicating areas of infarction.

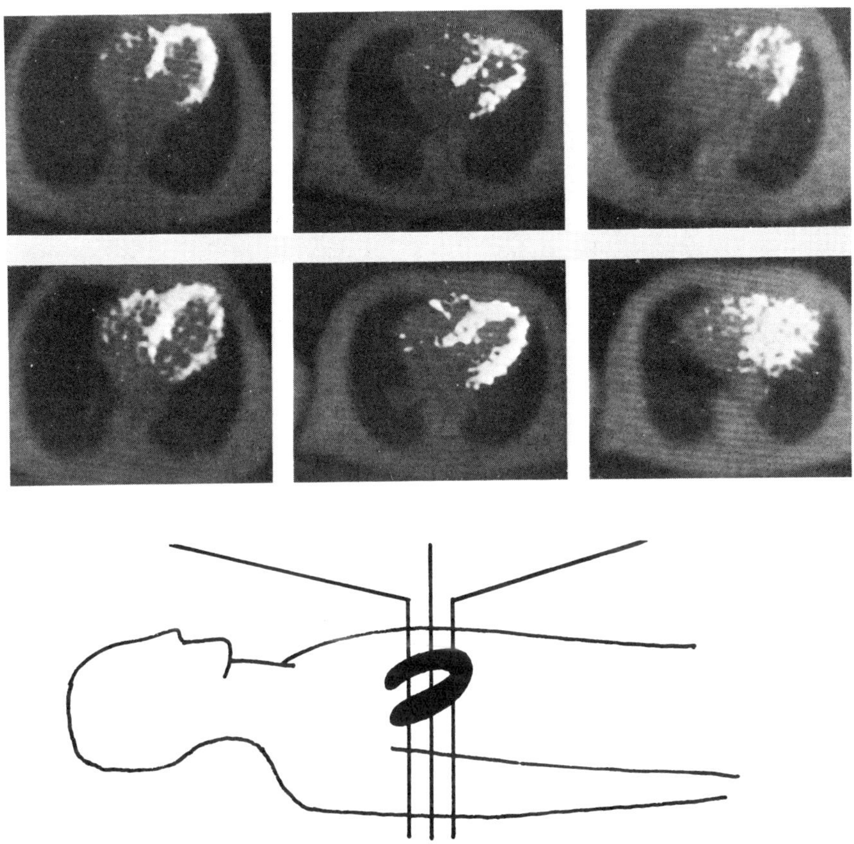

Figure 9. Rubidium-82 studies of coronary bypass patients.

Patient B had a perfusion defect in the upper section. Quantitative information of myocardial blood flow can be obtained if the input function (the amount of radioactivity in the blood that is delivered to the tissue) is obtained. This can be done from drawing regions of interest in the blood pool and the myocardium as shown in Figure 10. The computer extracted data from the PET images provides a graphical and quantitative output for the moment to moment changes of Rb-82 activity in the regions of interest (25,28).

Brain Studies. Rubidium-82 has also been used to study blood brain barrier changes in patients with brain tumors or Alzheimer's type senile dementia (28-30). The method of study is similar to the heart studies without gating. Figure 11 shows the uptake of Rb-82 in the three levels of a brain tumor. This non-invasive procedure provides information on the size and vascularity of the tumor. In the slice OM + 10 there is a vascular rim and a necrotic center in the tumor. The metabolism of glucose was determined in the same tumor patient using ^{18}F-fluorodeoxyglucose produced on a cyclotron and the results correlated well with Rb-82 distribution.

Summary

Automated radionuclide generators capable of providing precise dose delivery of multi-millicurie amounts of short-lived positron emitters on demand from a safe and easily operated system are an attractive alternative to on-site cyclotrons for positron emission tomography. The availability of curie quantities of parent radionuclides from national laboratories and the development of microprocessor automation makes it feasible to utilize these generators in the clinical setting.

We have demonstrated the use of generator produced Rb-82 as a readily available supply of a positron emitter for PET studies. At the same time, regional suppliers of cyclotron produced positron emitters can provide on a scheduled basis metabolic substrates such as ^{18}F-fluorodeoxyglucose by taking advantage of the 110 min half life of ^{18}F. Other applications of the Rb-82 generator are; the use of Rb-82 and 2.0 min oxygen-15 labeled H_2O in dual tracer kinetic studies to obtain information on coronary blood flow, pulmonary edema, extravascular lung water (31), and the intracoronary use of Rb-82 in the single photon mode with a rotating tungsten collimator to assess myocardial blood flow (32). The use of the constant infusion method to achieve steady state conditions for the measurement of myocardial blood flow has already been discussed as a method for using slower imaging systems.

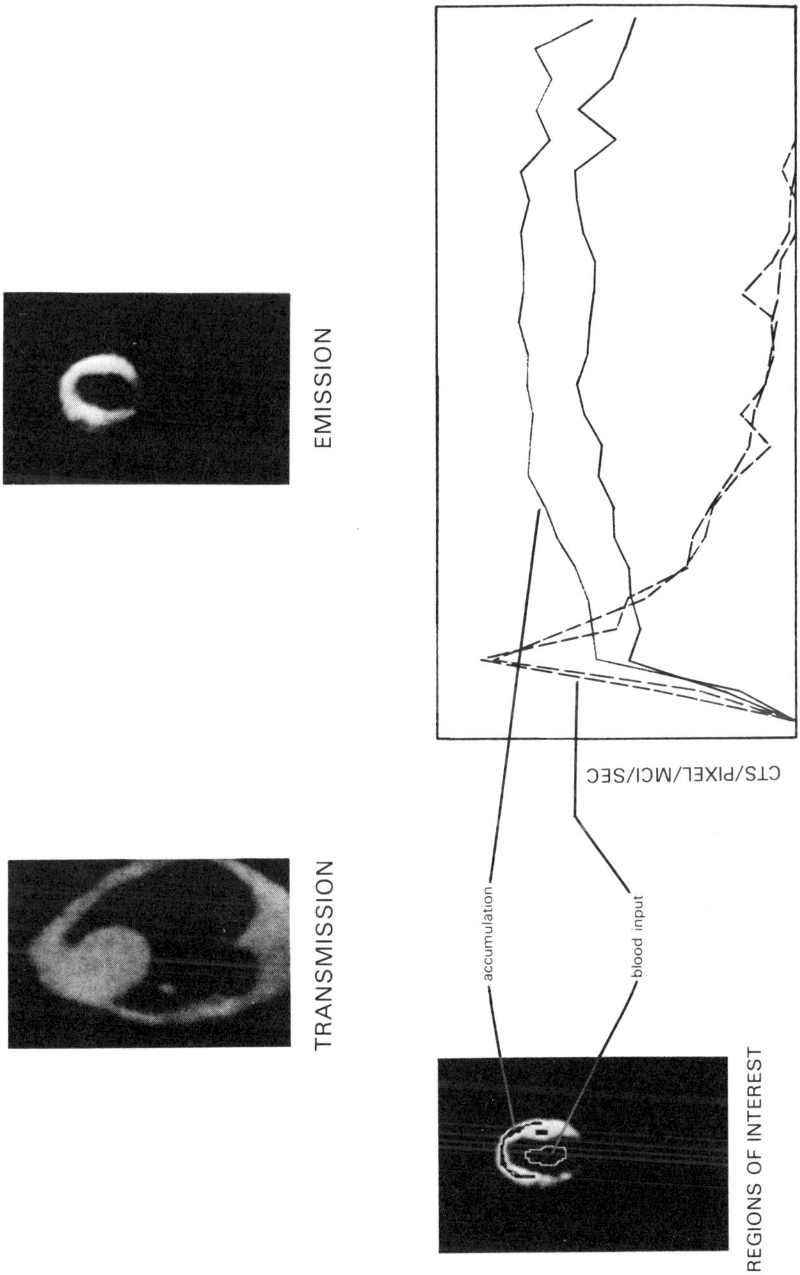

Figure 10. Measuring myocardial blood flow by the rubidium flow method.

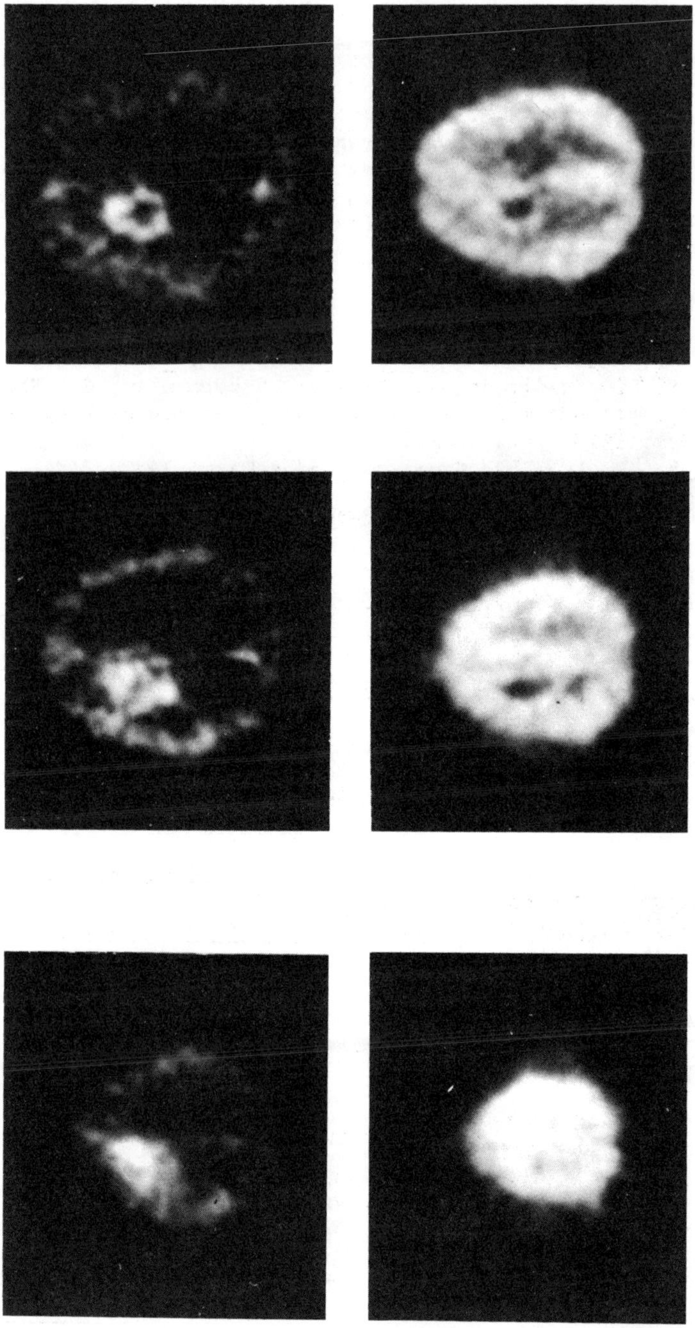

Figure 11. Rb-82 and F-18-fluorodeoxyglucose PET studies in a brain tumor patient.

Acknowledgments

This work was supported by DOE Contract No. DE-AC03-76SF00098 and NIH Grant No. 8605-53.

The authors thank M.S. Singh and W. P. Hemphill for technical assistance and D. C. Morris for preparation of the manuscript. The Sr-82 used in these studies was provided by Dr. H. A. O'Brien of Los Alamos Scientific Laboratory and the Ge/Li gamma analysis was done by Dr. C. T. Schmidt of Lawrence Berkeley Laboratory.

Literature Cited

1. Yano, Y.; Anger, H. O. J. Nucl. Med. 1968, 9, 2-6.
2. Yano, Y. in "Radiopharmaceuticals;" Subramanian, G., Rhodes, B.A.; Cooper, J. F.; Sodd, V.J. Eds.; Society of Nucl. Med., New York, 1975; pp. 236-245.
3. Yano, Y. J. Labelled Cpds. and Radiopharm. 1982, XIX, 1441-43.
4. Welch, M. J.; Thakur, M. L.; Coleman, R. E.; Patel, M. P.; Siegel, B. A.; Ter-Pogossian, M. M. J. Nucl. Med., 1977, 18, 558-62.
5. Hnatowich, D. J.; Layne, W. W.; Childs, R. L. Intl. J. Appl. Radiat. Isot. 1982, 33, 327-32.
6. Lagunas-Solar, M. C.; Little, F. E.; Moore, H. A. in Proc. Fourth Intl. Symp. Radiopharmaceutical Chemistry, 1982, 179-81.
7. Ku, T. H.; Richards, P.; Stang, L. G.; Prach, T. J. Nucl. Med., 1979, 20, 682.
8. Hui, J. C. K.; Atkins, H. L.; Som, P.; Ku, T. H.; Fairchild, R. G.; Giwa, L. O.; Richards, P. J. Nucl. Med., 1979, 20, 648.
9. Wisenberg, G.; Schelbert, H.; Robinson, G.; Selin, C.; Hoffman, E.; Phelps, M. J. Nucl. Med. 1979, 20, 648.
10. Richards, P.; Ku, T. H. Int. J. Appl. Radiat. Isot., 1979, 30, 250-254.
11. Braun, G.; Shulgin. A. T.; Sargent II, T. J. Labelled Compd. Radiopharm. 1978, 14, 767-773.
12. Yano, Y.; Anger, H. O. J. Nucl. Med. 1968, 9, 412-15.
13. Grant, P. M.; Erdal, B. R., O'Brien, H. A. J. Nucl. Med. 1975, 16, 300-4.
14. Yano, Y.; Roth, E. P. Intr. J. Appl. Radiat. Isot. 1979, 30, 382-85.
15. Yano, Y.; Budinger, T. F.; Chiang, G.; O'Brien, H. A.; Grant, P. M. J. Nucl. Med. 1979, 20, 961-6.
16. Kulprathipanja, S.; Hnatowich, D. I.; Beh, R. Intl. J. Appl. Radiat. Isot. 1979, 30, 447-9.
17. Horlock, P. L.; Clark, J. C., Goodier, I. W.; Barnes, J. W.; Bentley, G. E.,; Grant, P. M., O'Brien, H. A. J. Radional. Chem. 1981, 64, 257-265.

18. Vallabhajosula, S.; Cochavi, S.; Goldsmith, S. J.; Lipsye, H.; O'Brien, H. A. J. Nucl. Med. 1981, 22, p. 76.
19. Neirinckx, R. D.; Loberg, M. D. J. Nucl. Med. 1981, 22, p. 76.
20. Neirinckx, R. D.; Kronauge, J. F.; Gennaro, G. P.; Loberg, M. D. J. Nucl. Med. 1981, 22, 245-9.
21. Yano, Y.; Cahoon, J. L.; Budinger, T. F. J. Nucl. Med. 1981, 22, 1006-10.
22. Grant, P. M.; O'Brien, H. A., Jr.; Kahn, M. J. Inorg. Nucl. Chem. 1975, 37, 413-17.
23. Selwyn, A. P.; Allan, R. M.; L'Abbate, A.; Horlock, P.; Camici, P.; Clark, J.; O'Brien, H. A., Grant, P. M. Am. J. Cardiology, 1982, 50, 112-21.
24. Hoop, Jr., B.; Beh, R. A.,; Budinger, T. F. Chu, P.; Yano, Y.; Barnes, J. W. IEEE Trans. Nucl. Sci., 1976, NS-23, 584-589.
25. Budinger, T. F.; Derenzo, S. E.; Huesman, R. H.; in "Frontiers in Nuclear Medicine," Horst, W.; Wagner, H. N., Jr., Eds.; Springer-Verlag, Berlin, 1980, pp. 52-70.
26. Derenzo, S. E.,; Budinger, T. F.; Huesman, R. H.; Cahoon, J. L.; Vuletich, T. IEEE Trans. Nucl. Sci., 1981, NS-28(1), 81-89.
27. Budinger, T. F.; Yano, Y.; Derenzo, S. E.; Huesman, R. H.; Cahoon, J. L.; Mayer, B. R.; Greenberg, W. L.; O'Brien, Jr., H. A. J. Nucl. Med. 1979, 20, 603.
28. Budinger, T. F.; Yano, Y.; Mayer, B. R.; Mathis, C. A.; Ganz, E.; Huesman, R. H.; Derenzo, S. E. in "Proc. 3rd World Congress Nucl. Med. and Biology," Raynaud, C.; Ed., Pergamon Press, Paris, 1982, Vol. III, pp. 2238-41.
29. Yen, C. K.; Yano, Y.; Budinger, T. F.; Friedland, R. P.; Derenzo, S. E.; Huesman, R. H. J. Nucl. Med. 1982, 23, 532-37.
30. Friedland, R. P.; Yano, Y.; Budinger, T. F.; Ganz, E.; Huesman, R. H.; Derenzo, S. E.; Knittel, B. Euro. Neurology, 1983, 22, Suppl. 2, p. 19.
31. Tsui, B. M. W.; Bilfinger, T. V.; Fueltz, K. R.; Harper, P. V. J. Nucl. Med. 1982, 23, p. 74.
32. Harper, P. V.; Rujan, J. W.; Al-Sadir, J.; Chua, K. G.; Resnekov, L.; Neirinckx, R.; Loberg, M. J. Nucl. Med. 1982, 23, p. 69.

RECEIVED August 19, 1983

8

Large-Scale Isolation of Sr-82 for Generator Production

K. E. THOMAS and J. W. BARNES

Group INC-3, Los Alamos National Laboratory, Los Alamos, NM 87545

A new chemical separation process has been developed at Los Alamos for the isolation of Sr-82 from irradiated molybdenum targets. Large (up to 500 gram) molybdenum metal targets are irradiated for approximately one month at the Los Alamos Meson Physics Facility (LAMPF). Following irradiation, a no-carrier-added radiochemically pure strontium fraction is obtained from a chemical separation process involving one or two ion exchange columns. The new process is simpler to perform and results in a purer product than the process used in the past. This new procedure has been used in the production of up to 28 Curies of Sr-82 at end-of-bombardment. The product will be made available for commercial production of the Sr-82/Rb-82 generator system for medical use.

The Medical Radioisotope Research Group (INC-3) at Los Alamos National Laboratory has produced Sr-82 for use in collaborative experiments for several years. This has generally been from small (<150 g) molybdenum targets used for Br-77 production. Several of our collaborators have used our product for assessment of Sr-82/Rb-82 generator systems (1-3). Recently, E. R. Squibb and Sons, Inc., has expressed interest in obtaining larger quantities of Sr-82 for generator production. A goal of the studies reported here was to improve the purity of the Sr-82 product since, prior to this work, the strontium product was usually contaminated. This prompted a review of the chemical separation process then in use and the development of the process described in this paper.

The earlier method for isolation of Sr-82 (4), illustrated in Figure 1, involved three ion exchange columns, one solvent extraction, evaporations, and dilutions. On a small non-routine scale, this procedure was satisfactory. On a large scale, routine basis,

0097-6156/84/0241-0123$06.00/0
© 1984 American Chemical Society

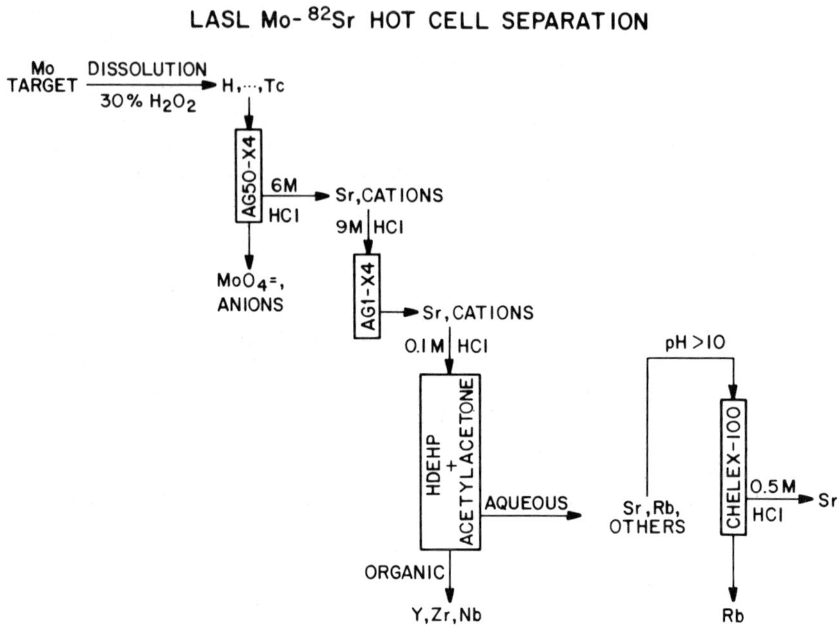

Figure 1. Flow scheme for the earlier strontium process.

the number of manipulations and the time involved becomes cumbersome. Typically, radioactive contaminants would include Mn-52, Mn-54, and Y-88, at higher than desired levels. This procedure was not designed for removal of manganese since this was never considered to be a problem; however, the extraction step was included to remove Y-88. The Y-88 problem was probably a result of entrainment and cross-contamination of phases in the extraction. Reevaluation of the process brought to mind alternative purification methods that should not only yield a clean product, but also be simpler to run.

The new chemistry is based on a Sr-90/Y-90 separation using α-hydroxyisobutyric acid (α-HIB) and cation exchange chromatography (5). Once the activities are loaded onto the column, the steps to prepare the column for the α-HIB elution remove several of the possibile contaminants including rubidium and cobalt. Finally, the α-HIB elution also removes a wide range of other elements as well, leaving strontium on the ion exchange column (6).

Experimental

Targets. The target consists of stacks of 0.25-0.50 mm thick molybdenum metal disks. One of several configurations is used depending on the quantity of Sr-82 desired. Various combinations of up to three stacks 2.5-cm and 1.9-cm in diameter with a thickness of 1.25 cm may be used to give target masses of 60 to 170 grams. Larger mass targets termed "big molys," may be prepared using 6.4-cm diameter stacks with thicknesses of 1.25 cm to 1.9 cm. Targets as great as 460 grams have been prepared in this manner.

Target packaging is illustrated in Figure 2, which shows two 1.9-cm and one 2.5-cm diameter stacks, 1.25-cm thick, held together with copper rings. The stacks are enclosed in a screwed-shut can to protect the target from the cooling water. The can is then contained inside the target carrier. This entire package is attached to the end of a stringer for irradiation.

Irradiations. The irradiations are performed at the Isotope Production Facility (IPF) at the Los Alamos Meson Physics Facility (LAMPF). Target handling has been described elsewhere (7-9). Irradiation lengths vary from 2 to 29 days at a nominal beam intensity of 500 μ-amps (at the IPF). Generally, the targets are located in irradiation positions (stringers) 2 or 3.

Chemistry. A flow chart of the new strontium process is shown in Figure 3. The dissolution procedures are the same as described for the Br-77 process (10). The HNO_3-H_3PO_4 dissolution is performed if Br-77 is to be recovered; otherwise, H_2O_2 is used for the dissolution. The HNO_3-H_3PO_4 dissolving solution is composed

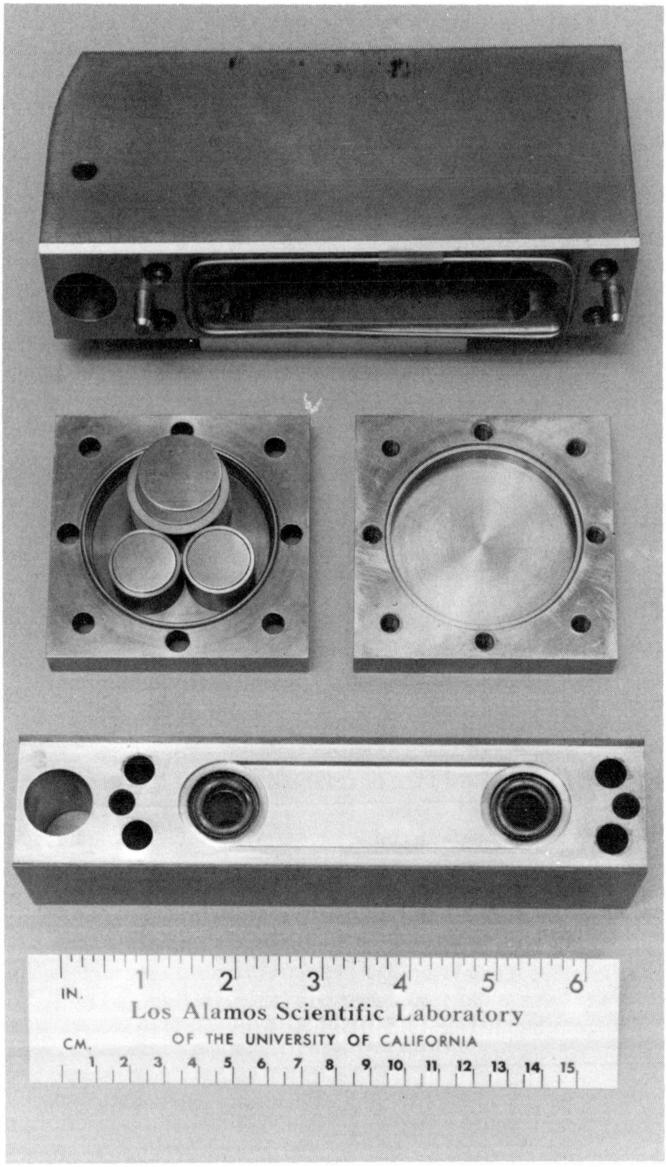

Figure 2. Target arrangement and packaging for a three-stack molybdenum metal target.

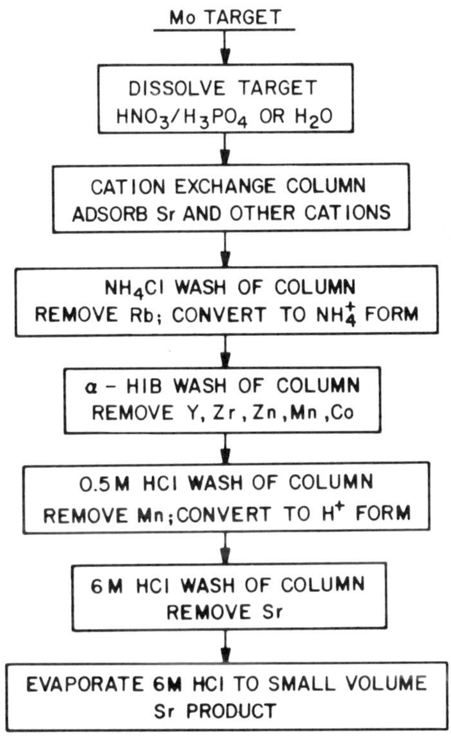

Figure 3. Flow scheme for the new strontium process. If H_2O_2 was used to dissolve the target, an anion exchange column in 12 M HCl is required to remove zirconium from the strontium product.

of 550 ml conc. HNO_3, 250 ml conc. H_3PO_4, and 200 ml H_2O. One liter of this solution has been used to dissolve as much as 170 grams of molybdenum metal. This solution is diluted with an equal volume of dioxane prior to the separation procedure. A second procedure uses 30% H_2O_2 as a dissolving solution; five liters of H_2O_2 have been used to dissolve about 300 g of the metal.

Once all the metal has been dissolved, the solution is passed through a cation exchange column (AG 50W-X8, 100-200 mesh; BioRad Laboratories). A bed volume of as little as 40 ml has been used successfully in this work. The resin removes the cations present from the large quantity of molybdate and any other anions that might be present. The column is now converted to the ammonium form by passing 0.5 M NH_4Cl through the column until the pH of the effluent is the same as the feed solution (∿pH 4.5). Next, approximately five column volumes of 0.5 M α-HIB (pH 4.5-5.0) are passed through the column. The α-HIB is now removed from the column via an H_2O wash. To convert the column back to the hydrogen form, about five column volumes of 0.5 M HCl are used. Finally, strontium is removed from the column with 6 M HCl.

If HNO_3-H_3PO_4 was used in the dissolution, the strontium product is radiochemically pure and is evaporated to dryness, dissolved in H_2O, and then strontium activity is determined for eventual shipping. If H_2O_2 was used, the product contains some zirconium and is taken to dryness, dissolved in concentrated HCl, and loaded onto an anion exchange column (AG 1X8, 100-200 mesh; BioRad Laboratories). This ion exchange step must be performed very soon after the first column due to growth of Y-88 from the zirconium contamination. Strontium passes through the anion column; this solution is evaporated to dryness, dissolved in H_2O and prepared for shipment.

Data Analysis. All samples are analyzed for radioactive nuclides by a Ge(Li)-pulse height analyzer system calibrated for counting 5-ml solution samples. In all cases, appropriate dilutions are made to reduce the activity level of the counting sample so that counting system dead-time is less than 15%. Gamma peak intensities are determined using a modified version of the peak fitting program GAMANAL (11). Individual nuclides are determined by identification of their associated gamma radiations. No half-life measurements are made as part of the identification process.

Results

Listed in Table I are the results of nine production runs for strontium. Targets ranging in mass from 64 to 457 grams have been irradiated with production as high as 28 Ci at end-of-bombardment

(EOB). Run number 30-1-2 was processed several months after EOB; this allowed observation of Sr-82 in the dissolved target solution. Normally this is not possible due to the large number of other nuclides present shortly after irradiation, several of which have the same gamma ray energy as Sr-82. Measurement of Sr-82 in the target solution of run 30-1-2 allowed an estimation of the strontium overall chemical yield. This was determined to be $\geq$90%. The overall yield on some of the later runs was roughly estimated to be 50-75%. In these studies some strontium yield was sacrificed to insure a pure final product and to shorten the time involved in preparing the sample for shipping.

The ratio of Sr-82 to Sr-85 at EOB is also shown in Table I. The Sr-83 to Sr-82 ratio has been determined for the last three runs. This ratio was determined to be 7.2, 6.5, and 3.0 for runs 33-1-14, -18, and -21, respectively.

The times required for the various procedure steps are given in Table II. The dissolution takes as long as three hours no matter which technique is used. Solution and column preparation time is roughly three hours and clean-up and waste disposal take about four hours.

Table I. Production of Sr-82

Run No.	μA-hr	Hours in Beam	Target Mass	Total Ci Sr-82 at EOB	Ratio at EOB 82/85
30-1-2	2.27×10^5	654	457	24.0	1.16
33-1-1	1.92×10^4	47	166	1.1	1.28
33-1-3	2.24×10^5	569	334	28.0	∿1.00
33-1-4	1.16×10^5	∿350	166	9.6	1.12
33-1-9	3.16×10^5	677	64	∿12.0	1.13
33-1-13	1.60×10^5	403	450	*	1.06
33-1-14	5.18×10^4	142	64	1.7	1.38
33-1-18	4.92×10^4	125	167	5.1	1.43
33-1-21	4.08×10^5	695	289	20.0	1.05

*Not all of target dissolved.

Discussion

The 0.5 M NH_4Cl wash of the ion exchange column is a good decontamination step for rubidium radioisotopes and also removes some cobalt and vanadium. Often, the ammonium chloride and the α-HIB solutions appear blue-green which probably results from massive amounts of copper from the target packaging. Both of these column

Table II. Time Requirements for the New Strontium Process

Step	Time Required (hours)
Dissolution	$\sim$3
Cation Column	$\leq$5
Evaporation	1-2
Anion Column	$\sim$2
Evaporation	0.5

washes remove all indications of large quantities of metal contaminants. The α-HIB elution was chosen specifically for removal of yttrium radioisotopes. This eluant also removes manganese, zinc, cobalt, vanadium, and copper, but zirconium is only partially removed. We have found that zirconium is not adsorbed onto the cation exchange column from the HNO_3-H_3PO_4 solution, but is at least partially adsorbed from H_2O_2.

In order for the yttrium elution to work properly, the pH must be maintained at greater than pH 4. This is accomplished by converting the column to the ammonium form. Otherwise, the pH of the α-HIB will decrease on the column and yttrium will not elute. After yttrium is eluted, the ammonium ion must be displaced from the column to prevent excessive salts in the final product. This is the reason for the 0.5 M HCl wash of the column after the α-HIB has been removed. The strontium product is obtained in 6 M HCl. Using a 40-50 ml resin bed, the strontium is obtained in a volume of approximately 100 ml. Some yield is sacrificed to keep this volume as small as possible to reduce the evaporation time.

The cation exchange resin AG MP-50 (BioRad Laboratories) was used for one run, 33-1-9, in anticipation of a greater separation factor for the yttrium-strontium separation. However, the column retained strontium, only slowly releasing it in 6 M-12 M HCl. A possible explanation is that strontium ions are adsorbed on the resin inside the large resin pores. When strong acid is passed over the resin, the pores contract, trapping the strontium ions within them. Because of the slow elution of strontium from this resin, AG MP-50 will not be used in the future for strontium purification.

As mentioned earlier, if H_2O_2 is used for the dissolution, some zirconium remains as a contaminant in the strontium fraction from the cation exchange column. This requires the additional anion exchange column and an extra evaporation which requires extra time. The cation exchange column has taken up to five hours to run. About half of this time is required for passing the dissolved target solution through the column. An additional one to two hours is required for the evaporation of the 100 ml of 6M HCl. If the anion exchange column is needed, a further two hours is required. A dissolution time of approximately three hours applies to both the H_2O_2 and HNO_3-H_3PO_4 cases and is performed the day prior to running the columns. However, Br-77 is usually produced for shipment from the HNO_3-H_3PO_4 dissolution and this solution can still be used for strontium production so that the dissolving time here is incidental to strontium production.

The new separation procedure is a major improvement. The number of manipulations of a strontium-containing solution has been reduced thus reducing the possibility of loss due to spillage and transfers. Also, the purity of the product has been greatly improved and is consistent. In all but two cases, no radioactive contaminants have been observed in the final product. In one of those exceptions, the ion exchange bed was damaged and, in the other, a small amount of Y-87 was observed at a moderate level. An additional improvement has been the chemical yield. From early runs, experience led us to expect about one-third of the actual amount recovered from the new process. From this and the fact that we had obtained 90% yield from the new process, we estimate the chemical yield of the old process to be roughly 30%.

In Table III, the specifications we require on our final product are summarized. This process is performed on a "no carrier added" level. The only strontium present in the final sample is that produced in the nuclear reaction and introduced as an impurity in the target and reagents. Usually the concentration of Sr-82 in the final product is on the order of a factor of ten higher than that listed in the table. When the minimum concentration is approached, the volume to be shipped becomes unreasonably large. We do not check the actual acid concentration of the final product. As described earlier, the 6 M HCl is taken to dryness and then brought up in H_2O. There is enough residual HCl in the evaporation flask to make the solution slightly acidic. All shipments made since January 1982 have met the radionuclidic purity characteristics. Even in the two exceptions to the pure strontium fractions, the Y-87 did not exceed 0.005 mCi/mCi Sr-82 at time of shipping.

No radionuclidic contaminants of other elements have been observed in the shipped material. Of course, Sr-85 is always present and Sr-83 is present at short intervals after the irradiation. The presence of Sr-83 in the product leads to the formation of Rb-83 in the eluant from the generator. Large quantities of Sr-85 cause problems in shielding the generator. Inspection of the production data allows one to make the following characterizations of the strontium product: a) for short irradiations ($\sim$200 hours), the 82/85 ratio at EOB averages approximately 1.4 and the

Table III. Characteristics of The Final Strontium Product

Specific Activity	No Carrier Added
Concentration of Sr-82	>50 mCi/ml
Chemical Form	Dilute HCl
Radionuclidic Purity*:	
Sr-85	≤5 mCi/mCi Sr-82
Sr-83	<0.04 mCi/mCi Sr-82
Rb-83	<0.15 mCi/mCi Sr-82
All Other	<0.01 mCi/mCi Sr-82

*At time of shipment.

83/82 ratio at EOB is roughly 6.9; b) for long irradiations (>200 hours), the 82/85 ratio at EOB is about 1.1 and the 83/82 ratio (from one measurement) at EOB is 3.0. Figure 4 illustrates the change in the 82/85 and 83/82 ratios versus time after EOB. The "worst" cases of EOB ratios of 82/85 of 1.1 and 83/82 of 6.9 have been chosen for illustration. This graph shows a usable lifetime of at least 100 days after EOB for the strontium solution. The 83/82 limit would be reached, at most, about ten days after EOB. Chemistry is usually performed 7 to 14 days after EOB and at least two days elapse before shipment to the users. A problem has been the detection of Sr-83. Prior to the last three runs, chemistry was performed 14 days or more after EOB. Shown on the graph is our estimated detection limit of 0.006 mCi/mCi Sr-82, which is reached at about 14 days after EOB explaining why Sr-83 had not been observed from earlier runs.

Summary

A new production procedure for Sr-82 has been developed which requires less time and effort than the previously used procedure. It also consistently yields a product meeting a strict set of specifications. The preferred method of dissolution, HNO_3-H_3PO_4, allows the entire purification to be performed on one cation exchange column.

The final strontium product has a useable lifetime of at least 100 days after EOB. It should satisfy the 83/82 limit within 10 days after EOB. It is possible to produce as much as 28 Ci of Sr-82 (at EOB) from a single irradiation using the "big moly" targets. If smaller quantities are desired, smaller targets and shorter irradiation times may be used for production of curie quantities of Sr-82 as well as Br-77.

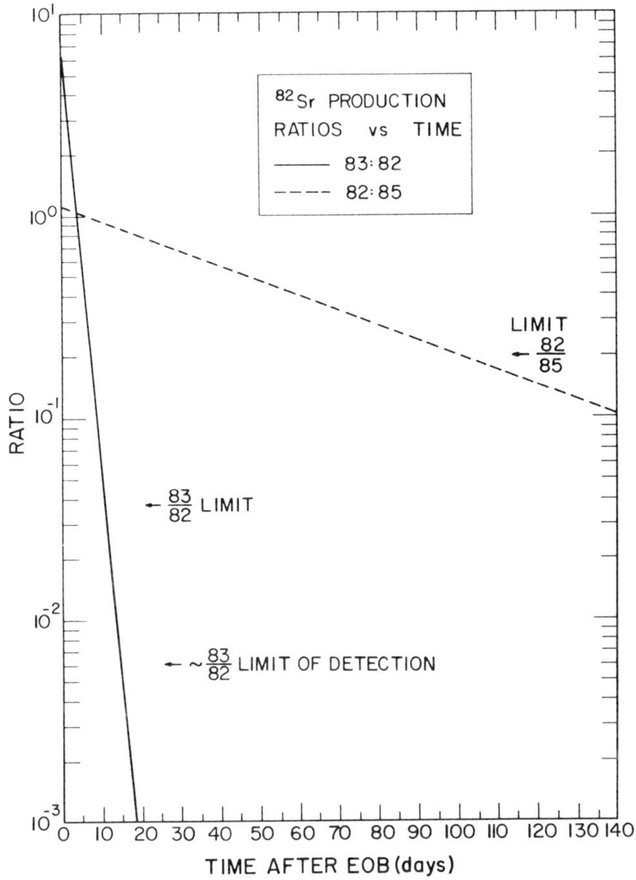

Figure 4. Change in ratios versus time after EOB for the strontium isotope ratios 82:85 and 83:82. "Limit" refers to the radionuclidic requirements listed in Table III.

Acknowledgments

The authors wish to thank M. A. Ott and F. H. Seurer for the target preparation and the irradiations, and W. Taylor for assistance in the earlier tests of the chemistry.

Literature Cited

1. Neirinckx, R. D.; Kronange, J. F.; Gennaro, G. P.; Loberg, M.D. J. Nucl. Med. 1982, 23, 245-249.
2. Yano, Y.; Budinger, T. F.; Chiang, G.; O'Brien, H. A.; Grant, P. M. J. Nucl. Med. 1979, 20, 961-966.
3. Grant, P. M.; Whipple, R. E.; O'Brien, H. A.; Kulprathipanja, S. J. Nucl. Med. 1978, 19, 1250-1255.
4. Bentley, G. E.; Barnes, J. W.; Grant, P. M.; Whipple, R. E.; Wanek, P. M.; Ott, M. A.; DeBusk, T. P.; O'Brien, H. A. Am. Chem. Soc./Chem. Soc. Japan Chem Congress Abst. of Papers, Part 1, 1979, NUCL-33.
5. Bryant, E. A.; Sattizahn, J. E.; Warren, B. Am. Chem. Soc. 133rd Meeting, 1958.
6. Thomas, K. W.; Prestwood, R. J., personal communication.
7. Cummings, C. E.; Ogard, A. E.; Shaw, R. H. Proc. 26th Conf. Remote Systems Technology, 1978, pp. 201-206.
8. Bentley, G. E.; Barnes, J. W.; DeBusk, T. P.; Ott, M. A. Proc. 26th Conf. Remote Systems Technology, 1978, p. 378-381.
9. "Isotope Production Facility" in LAMPF Users Handbook, Los Alamos National Laboratory report MP-DO-1-UHB (Rev) 1980, 6B-7.
10. Grant, P. M.; Whipple, R. E.; Barnes, J. W.; Bentley, G. E.; Wanek, P. M.; O'Brien, H. A. J. Inorg. Nucl. Chem. 1981, 43, 2217-2222.
11. Gunnink, R.; Niday, J. B. Lawrence Livermore National Laboratory report UCRL-51061 (Vols. 1-4), 1971-1972.

RECEIVED September 11, 1983

9

A Radionuclide Generator and Infusion System for Pharmaceutical Quality Rb-82

G. P. GENNARO, R. D. NEIRINCKX, B. BERGNER, W. R. MULLER, A. WARANIS, T. A. HANEY, S. L. BARKER, M. D. LOBERG, and A. YARNAIS

The Squibb Institute for Medical Research, New Brunswick, NJ 08903

The short lived positron-emitter Rb-82 (t 1/2=1.26m) has potential application in cardiovascular diagnostic nuclear medicine. A generator system containing the parent Sr-82 has been developed that will provide an eluate of Rb-82 suitable for direct infusion. The Rb-82 is eluted by a syringe pump from a hydrous stannic oxide column in a continuous stream of physiological saline solution. The rate of elution (infusion) can be controlled from 10 to 100 ml/min. At elution rates of 25, 50, and 75 ml/min, 100% of label potency (Rb-82 activity divided by Sr-82 activity X 100) is delivered in 47, 51, & 57 ml, respectively. At these same elution rates the peak of Rb-82 activity (bolus) emerges in 45 sec, 22 sec, and 15 sec, respectively. The breakthrough of Sr-82 is typically less than 1 x 10^{-5} uCi Sr-82/ml/mCi Rb-82 in 50 ml. A positron sensitive detector monitors and integrates the eluted activity. This instrument may be set to select any fraction of the eluate activity for administration and to terminate the delivery at any preset dose.

Rubidium-82 (t 1/2=1.26 min) is produced by electron capture decay of Sr-82 (t 1/2=25 days). As an alkali metal cation, the physiological behavior of rubidium is analagous to potassium and, therefore, has been considered as a diagnostic agent for myocardial perfusion studies. Benefits of Rb-82 over other radionuclides for diagnostic scintigraphy include reduced patient and personnel radiation exposure (1), a short half-life that permits rapid sequential imaging to evaluate the effects of intervention, and a decay scheme that permits full utilization of positron emission tomography. Rubidium-82 can be conveniently obtained on demand from a radionuclide generator system loaded with parent Sr-82, providing the radionuclidic separation is efficient enough to insure the absence of long-lived Sr-82 in the generator eluate.

0097-6156/84/0241-0135$06.00/0
© 1984 American Chemical Society

Previously reported Sr-82/Rb-82 generators have been based upon both organic (2) and inorganic (3,4) exchangers (Table I). Organic resins, such as Bio-Rex 70 and Chelex 100, are subject to radiolytic degradation which may reduce radiochemical separation efficiency and may produce chemical, and possibly pyrogenic, contaminants. Radiolytically stable inorganic exchangers are therefore preferred. The ideal Rb-82 generator would maintain low Sr-82 breakthrough at high elution rates with physiologic eluents. It must also provide a high yield of Rb-82 and be usable for large numbers of elutions. Drawbacks to many other promising systems included the need to maintain a high eluent pH and use of hypertonic eluent (4). Recent investigations (5,6) have focused attention on hydrous tin oxide as a suitable adsorbent for Sr-82. As with other hydrous metal oxides, such as alumina and zirconia, tin oxide is an amphoteric ion exchanger that exhibits cation exchange properties at basic pH. Hydrous tin oxide, however, appears to be particularly favored by virtue of its high Sr(II) distribution coefficient (Kd=Sr-bound/Sr-free) and high separation factor, Kd[Sr(II)/Rb(I)], over a broad pH range (Table II; Figure 1).

The potential yield of a Rb-82 generator is dictated by the nature of secular equilibrium. Thus, the activities of parent (Sr-82) and daughter (Rb-82) are nearly equivalent at equilibrium (Rb-82/Sr-82 = 1.00004). After separation of the Rb-82 by generator elution, equilibrium is re-established quickly. The fractional regeneration of daughter activity is given by (Eq. 1):

$$A(T)/A(eq) = (1-e^{-\lambda t}) \qquad (1)$$

where λ = decay constant for Rb-82. A Sr-82/Rb-82 generator is 75% recharged at 2.5 minutes and 95% recharged at 5.4 minutes. As a consequence of the short daughter half-life, generator yields are dependent on the eluent flow rate. For bolus elutions, maximum flow rate and minimum dead volume are required to minimize the loss of Rb-82 through decay during transit to the subject. In a continuous infusion mode, the extraction yield (and hence the attainable steady state infused radioconcentration) will increase with flow rate. A full discussion of elution kinetics for generator produced isotopes of short half-life has been given by Guillaume and Brihaye (7), who have observed that the clinically optimum flow rate will be that which delivers the minimum volume necessary to achieve an image of diagnostic value. This may be achieved at an intermediate, rather than at maximum, flow rate.

When dealing with a short-lived radionuclide generator, an infusion system will be needed for elution of the generator, recording of patient dose, and administration of the activity. The effective utilization of 76 sec Rb-82 will depend on its rapid extraction from the generator. Thus, the foremost feature of an infusion system will be the attainment of a high and uniform flow

Table II. Distribution Coefficients (Kd) of Sr(II) and Rb(I) (0.9% NaCl Solutions at 60 Min Equilibration).*

Adsorbent	pH	Sr(II)	Rb(I)	Sr(II)/Rb(I)
Basic alumina	8	7,000 ± 1,000	9 ± 2	800
Hydrous zirconium oxide	7	800 ± 100	5 ± 1	200
Hydrous titanium oxide	8	56,000 ± 9,000	56 ± 3	1,000
Titanium peroxide	7	43,000 ± 7,000	162 ± 3	300
Polyantimonic acid	3	75,000 ± 15,000	≤3	≥25,000
Hydrous tin oxide	7.2	53,000 ± 6,000	2.5 ± 1	21,000

*R. D. Neirinckx, J. F. Kronauge, and M. D. Loberg, Int. J. Appl. Radiat. Isotopes, 34: 721-25 (1983).

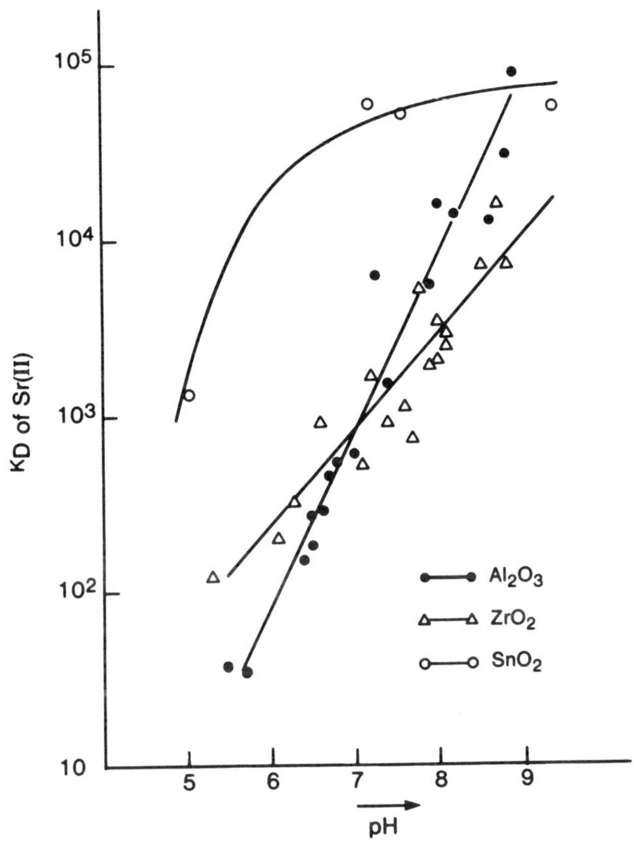

Figure 1. Strontium(II) distribution coefficients as a function of pH in 0.9% sodium chloride.

rate. Furthermore, other considerations in the design of an infusion system should include the following:

1. The pharmaceutical requirement to maintain eluate sterility and apyrogenicity,
2. Minimum dead volume of eluate tubing to reduce decay during administration,
3. Physical strength to withstand frequent use over long periods,
4. Control of volume and rate of delivery,
5. Real-time display of eluted activity and the means of terminating the infusion at a pre-set patient administered dose,
6. Choice of continuous or bolus infusion modes, and
7. Valving to divert low specific concentration eluate to "waste". Syringe delivery systems containing many of these features have been developed at the University of California (8-11), and this system is described in detail by Yano, Budinger, Cahoon and Huesman in their chapter in this volume.

We have developed and tested a Rb-82 infusion system that incorporates all of these features (Figure 2). The system is a mobile, self-contained pump, generator, and dosimeter (Figure 3). The electromechanical syringe pump can be set to deliver saline at any flow rate from 10 to 100 ml/minute. Saline is transferred through sterile tubing to a 150 ml sterile, disposable plastic syringe. Check valves at the syringe output automatically direct the eluent in either filling or infusion modes. The generator is connected to the system by sterile, PVC luer-lock tubing and is contained within a lead shield one and one half inches thick. The eluate activity is carried through PVC tubing past a radiation detector and through a two-way microprocessor controlled valve, which directs the eluate to either the subject or to a waste collection bottle, both of which terminate in a 0.22 μ sterilizing filter. The position of this valve is determined by the elution mode selected at the control module.

The infusion system may be set to elute the generator at any preset flow rate in any of the following modes:

1. Volume priority, in which the infusion will stop when the patient has received a preset volume (ml).
2. Dose priority, in which the infusion will stop when the patient has received a preset dose (mCi).
3. Bolus priority, in which the eluate is directed initially to the waste collection bottle until the onset of the bolus (adjustable onset level, mCi/sec) diverts the eluate stream to the patient line until the preset dose is accumulated.

Experimental

Generator Preparation. Strontium-82 is obtained from Los Alamos National Laboratory (LASL). The isotope is produced by a high energy spallation reaction on molybdenum and the purified mixture contains other strontium isotopes, notably Sr-83/Rb-83 and Sr-85.

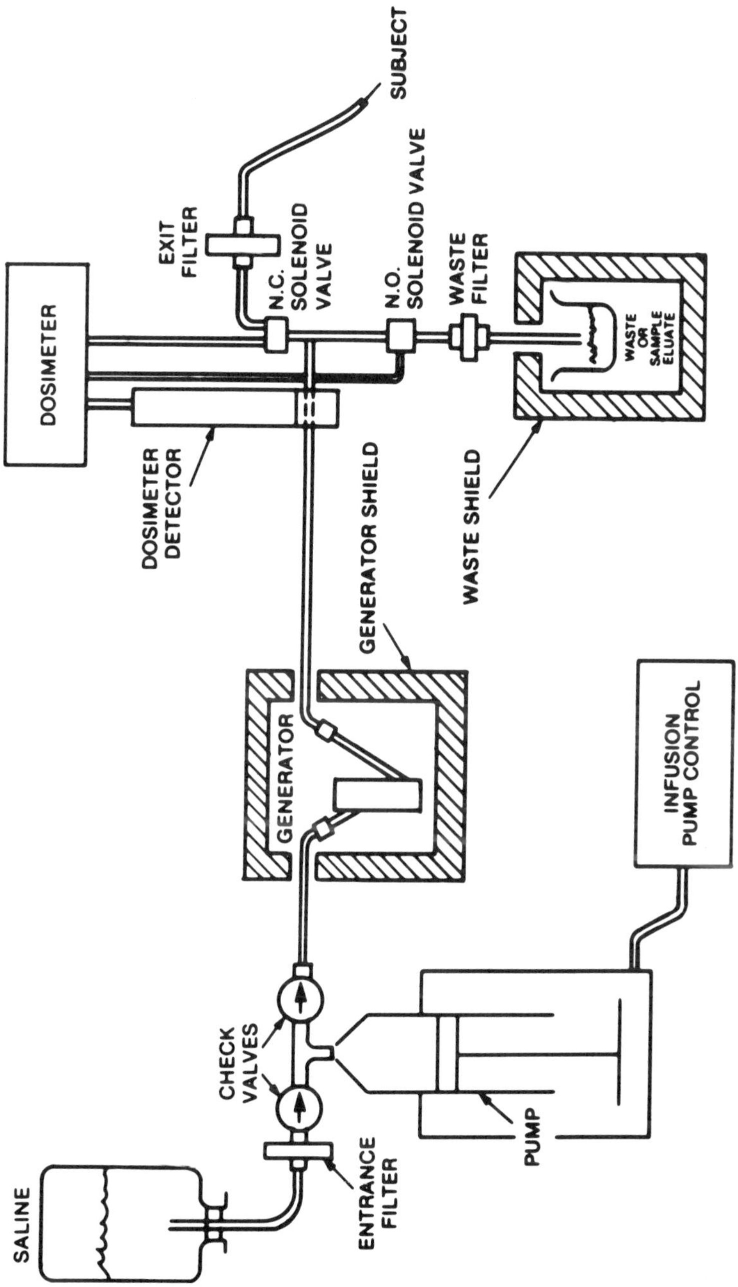

Figure 2. Block diagram of Rb-82 generator and infusion system.

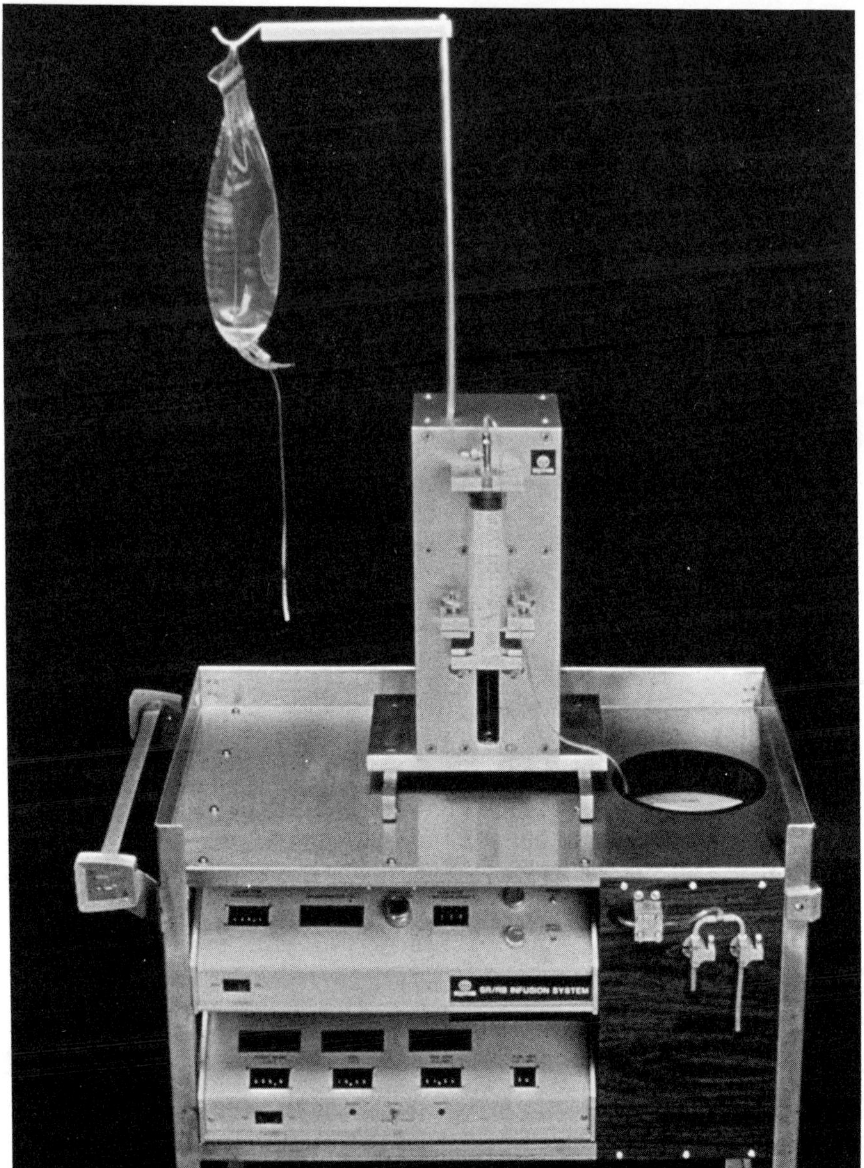

Figure 3. Mobile, self-contained infusion system for Rb-82 generator.

Radionuclidic analyses are performed with either a lithium-drifted germanium or intrinsic germanium detector. The assay for Sr-82 is based upon its 777 keV photon of 13.6% abundance. Strontium-85, which is often present in amounts comparable to that of Sr-82, is assayed by its 514 keV photopeak, which must be resolved from prominent 511 keV annihilation radiation by a curve stripping procedure (12).

Up to 150 mCi of Sr-82 (containing up to 300 mCi of Sr-85) is transferred to a column containing hydrous tin oxide. The column is washed with 0.9% sodium chloride to remove Rb-83 radiocontaminants. This column is fitted with luer-lock connectors to facilitate its use with sterile PVC tubing. The generator is eluted with 0.9% sodium chloride. The eluent is delivered by the syringe pump of the infusion system. Eluates are collected in 50 ml stoppered vials for nuclear and chemical analyses. Rb-82 may be conveniently measured in an ion chamber (dose calibrator). We have confirmed that the potentiometer setting recommended by the instrument manufacturer (Capintec, Montvale, NJ) is accurate. A sample of freshly eluted Rb-82 was measured by both a dose calibrator and, after suitable decay, a calibrated Ge(Li) spectrometer system. Data for both instruments lay along a single exponential decay of 76 sec half-life. Our evaluation of the Sr-82/Rb-82 generator performance is based primarily on measurement of yield, breakthrough, and elution profile.

Yield. The Rb-82 content of 50 ml of eluate, decay corrected to end of elution, collected at 50 ml/min is measured in a Capintec CRC-17 dose calibrator using the potentiometer setting recommended by the manufacturer for Rb-82. While this datum is not as significant as the dynamic yield information obtained from measurement of elution profiles, it is valuable in preliminary development work and in monitoring the performance of a given unit through an extended use period.

Breakthrough. Eluate radionuclidic purity is determined by NaI scintillation spectrometry on 50 ml of eluate. Samples must be held at least one hour before measurement to allow full decay of Rb-82. To improve sensitivity of measurement, the most prominent 511+514 keV peak is counted. Computations are based upon comparison with an aliquot of Sr-82+Sr-85 solution used to prepare the generator. Data are expressed in units of μCi Sr-82/ml of eluate/mCi Rb-82 at end of elution.

Elution Profile. Elution profiles are determined with the in-line radiation detector. For calibration of the in-line detector, equations developed for quantitative radiochromatography may be adapted. For a single detector, isotope, and geometry, which is in effect controlled by the tubing used to carry the eluate past the detector, a simple expression can be written (Eq. 2):

$$A = C \cdot F / K \qquad (2)$$

where A = the integrated activity in mCi; C = counts; F = flow rate of eluate in ml/min; and K = constant of proportionality. The flow rate term is kept independent of the proportionality constant to allow for separate adjustment of the flow rate without the need to readjust the calibration factor for the detector. Thus, the scalers on the dosimeter module may be set to display in mCi of Rb-82, since the circuit incorporates an adjustable pulse divider corresponding to the proportionality constant. In addition to displaying the activity of Rb-82 passing the detector at any instant, the second scaler provides a summation of total activity eluted. The flow rate constant, F, is set equal to the flow rate control of the infusion pump.

The calibration of the in-line detector is accomplished by comparing the end-of-elution collected dose (as measured in a dose calibrator) to the differential elution profile (as measured by the in-line detector). With data collection at 1 sec intervals, a 50 ml elution at 50 ml/min will produce 60 data points (N_i), each of which must be corrected to end-of-elution. The calibration factor for the in-line detector may be calculated from a single elution (Eq. 3) where EOE is the end of elution.

$$K = C \cdot F/A = \frac{\Sigma N_i \ e^{-\lambda t} \cdot F \text{ (ml/min)}}{\text{Rb-82 (mCi, EOE)}} \qquad (3)$$

Results and Discussion

The Rb-82 generators thus prepared were evaluated by repetitive, high volume elutions using the infusion system described earlier. Eluent was exclusively sterile, 0.9% sodium chloride solution with collections made into sterile, vented serum vials.

Yield. The Rb-82 content of 50 ml eluates collected at 50 ml/min is 71.7±6.5% of the Sr-82 potency of the generator. Frequent elutions over extended periods will slightly improve this value. After three weeks' elution with 2 liters of 0.9% sodium chloride, the collected end of elution yield will be 5-10% greater than initial yields.

Elution Profile. The differential elution profiles at three different flow rates are shown in Figure 4. As expected, the Rb-82 yield improves at faster flow rates with less activity being lost to decay. Integral outputs are shown in Figures 5 and 6. These values represent, respectively, the administered dose and the collected dose. The former data, which represent the integrated dosimeter readings of the on-line detector, must be considered in establishing the duration of infusion consistent with

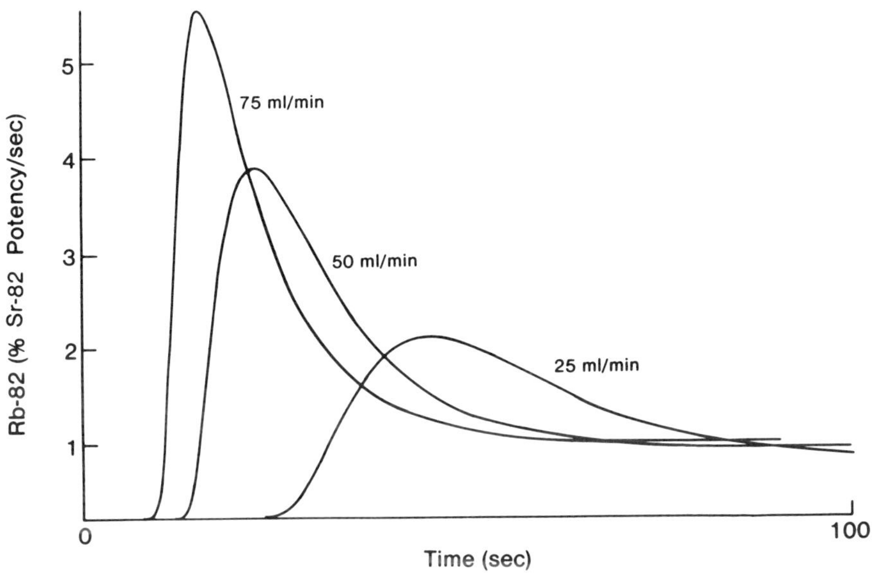

Figure 4. Elution profile of Rb-82 as a function of time for three selected flow rates.

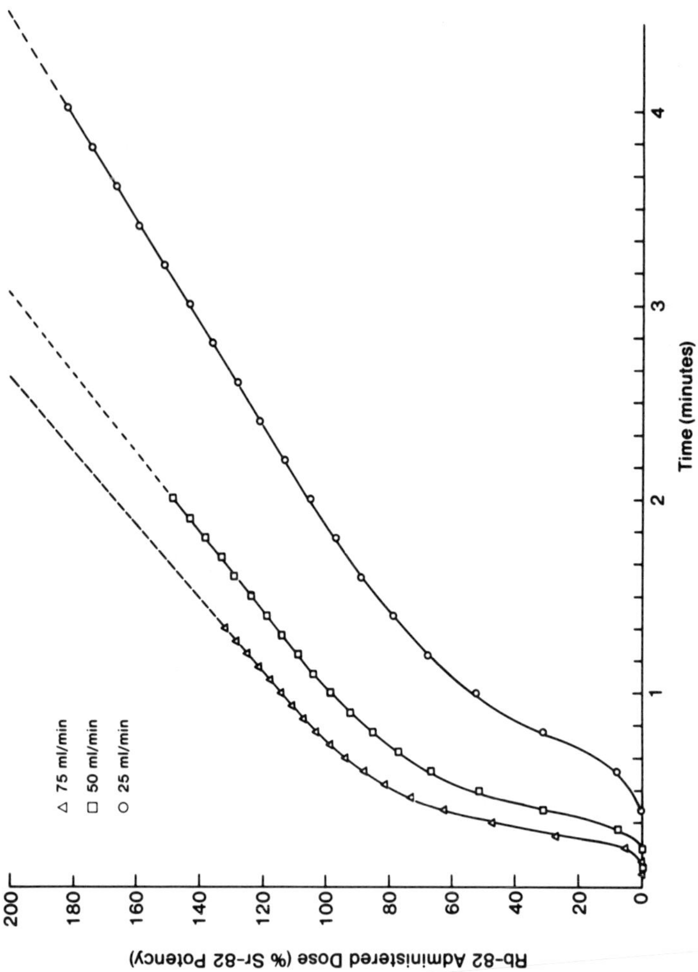

Figure 5. Total activity administered from a Rb-82 generator as a function of time for three selected flow rates.

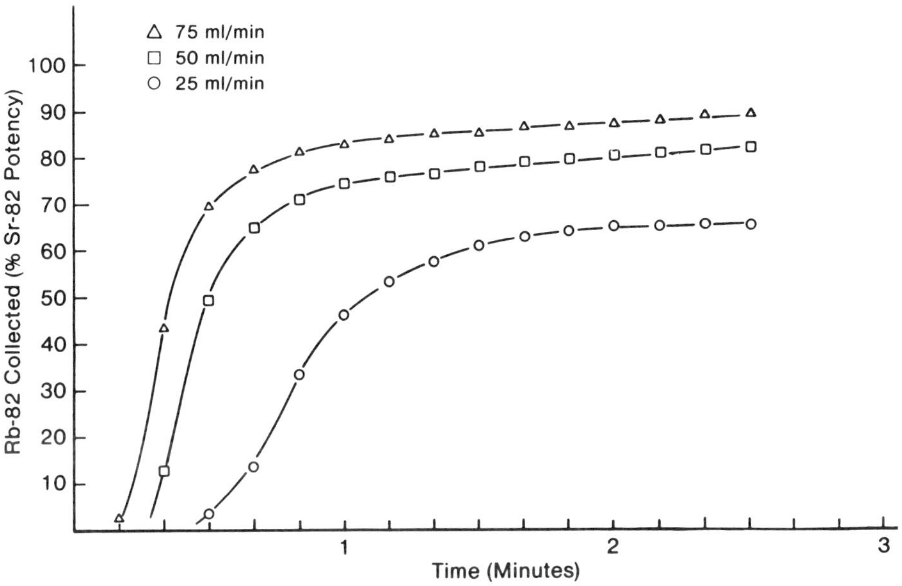

Figure 6. Steady-state administered activity from a Rb-82 generator as a function of time for three selected flow rates.

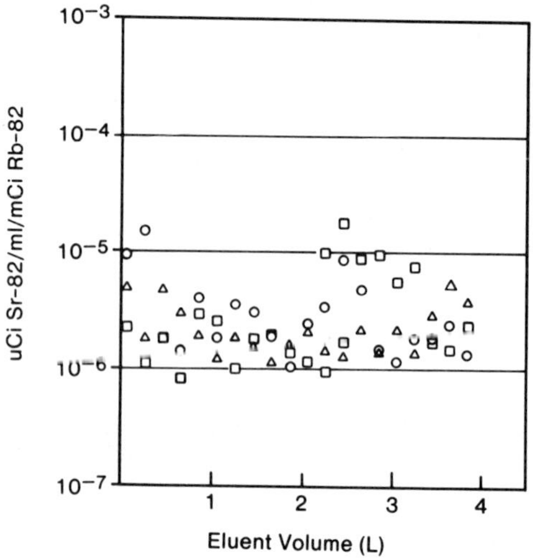

Figure 7. Strontium-82 breakthrough for elutions collected at 50 mL/min.

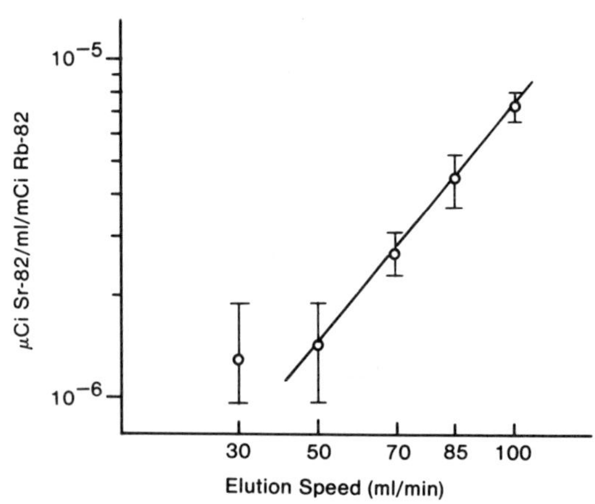

Figure 8. Strontium-82 breakthrough as a function of flow rate.

the patient absorbed dose. The latter data, which are decay corrected, indicate the in-vivo radioconcentration during the infusion. At a nominal flow rate of 50 ml/min, approximately 80% of the full generator potency will be available for diagnostic imaging.

Chemical Purity. Selected eluates from a 4 liter elution program were subjected to analyses for chemical and biological purity. At the end of four weeks of continued use, during which 4 liters of eluate were collected, samples were sterile and non-pyrogenic. Isotonicity was confirmed (NaCl = 8.94±.03 mg/ml) and neutrality maintained (pH = 6.27±0.16). No tin was detected in generator eluates by differential pulse polarography above a detection limit of 0.1 μg/ml. The radionuclidic identity of Rb-82 is easily confirmed by verification of its 76 sec half-life or through gamma spectrometry.

Breakthrough. Strontium-82 contamination of eluates from three generators is shown in Figure 7 for total elution volumes of 4 liters. Breakthrough is less than 1×10^{-5} μCi Sr-82/ml/mCi Rb-82 throughout the test period. Other generators have been eluted to total volumes of 20 liters, with no increase in breakthrough above 1×10^{-5} μCi Sr-82/ml/mCi Rb-82. Furthermore, low breakthrough levels are maintained up to flow rates of 100 ml/min (Figure 8).

Summary

The rubidium-82 eluate from this generator system is pharmaceutically suitable for direct venous infusion. Imaging may be based on positron emission tomography (13). Alternatively, images of diagnostic quality should be anticipated from single photon detection systems, provided that the instrumentation is compatable with these high energy photons. The feasibility of modifying conventional instruments for Rb-82 has been demonstrated by Ryan, et.al. (14) and Cochavi, et.al. (15). Thus Rb-82, as produced and administered by this system, may have potential clinical utility for myocardial perfusion (16), evaluation of brain tumors (13), and kidney imaging (15).

Literature Cited

1. Kearfott, K.J. J. Nucl. Med. 1982, 23, 1128-1132.
2. Yano, Y.; Roth, E. P. Int. J. Appl. Radiat. Isotopes 1979, 30, 382-385.
3. Kulprathipanja, S.; Hnatowich, D.J.; Beh, R. Int. J. Applied Radiat. Isotopes 1979, 30, 447-449.
4. Horlock, P.L.; Clark, J.C.; Goodier, I.W.; Barnes, J.W.; Bentley, G.E.; Grant, P.M.; O'Brien, H.A. J. Radioanal. Chem. 1981, 64, 257-265.

5. Neirinckx, R.D.; Kronauge, J.F.; Gennaro, G.P.; Loberg, M.D.; Los Alamos Medical Radioisotope Group, J. Nucl. Med. 1982, 23, 245-249.
6. Brihaye, Cl.; Guillaume, M.; Cogneau, M. Radiochem. Radioanal. Letters 1981, 48, 157-164.
7. Guillaume, M.; Brihaye, Cl. J. Biophys. Med. Nucl. 1982, 6, 137-142.
8. Yano, Y.; Anger, H.O. J. Nucl. Med. 1968, 9, 412-415.
9. Budinger, T.F.; Yano, Y.; Hoop, B. J. Nucl. Med. 1975, 16, 429-431.
10. Yano, Y.; Budinger, T.F.; Chiang, G.; O'Brien, H.A.; Grant, P.M. J. Nucl. Med. 1979, 20, 961-966.
11. Yano, Y.; Cahoon, J.L.; Budinger, T.F. J. Nucl. Med. 1981, 22, 1006-1010.
12. Waters, S.L.; Butler, K.R.: Clark, J.C.; Horlock, P.L.; Kensett, M.J.; Goodier, I.W.; Makepeace, J.; Smith, D.; Woods, M.J.; Barnes, J.W.; Bentley, G.E.; Grant, P.M.; O'Brien, H.A. Int. J. Appl. Radiat. Isotopes 1983, in press.
13. Yen, C.-K.; Yano, Y.; Budinger, T.F.; Friedland, R.P.; Derenzo, S.E.; Huesman, R.H.; O'Brien, H.A. J. Nucl. Med. 1982, 23, 532-537.
14. Chua, K.G.; Ryan, J.W.; Al-Sadir, J.; Resnekov, L.; Harper, P.V. IX World Congress of Cardiology, Moscow, June 20-26, 1982.
15. Neirinckx, R.D.; Cochavi, S.; Gennaro, GP.; Loberg, M.D.; Kronauge, J.F.; Goldsmith, S.L.; O'Brien, H.A. III World Congress of Nuclear Medicine and Biology, Paris, Aug. 29 - Sept. 2, 1982.
16. Budinger, T.F.; Yano, Y.; Derenzo, S.E.; Huesman, R.H.; Cahoon, J.L.; Moyer, B.R.; Greenberg, W.L.; O'Brien, H.A. J. Nucl. Med. 1979, 20, 603.

RECEIVED August 19, 1983

10

Evaluation of Adsorbents for the Ta-178 Generator

R. D. NEIRINCKX—Department of Radiology, Harvard Medical School, Boston, MA 02115

J. TRUMPER—Soreq Nuclear Research Center, Yavne, Israel

A. LEBLANC and P. C. JOHNSON—National Air and Space Administration, Life Sciences Division, Houston, TX 77058

The currently used Ta-178 generator is based on a radiation sensitive adsorbent and can be eluted about 50 times before W-178 breakthrough becomes unacceptable. We evaluated a series of inorganic and organic adsorbents as support for this generator. Hydrated inorganic materials adsorb tantalum very strongly from most aqueous solutions and none was found useful for the W-178/Ta-178 generator. Tantalum complexing agents are not able to desorb tantalum without dissolving the adsorbents to an appreciable extent. Chelating resins with a high affinity for W were investigated because they could reduce the W-178 breakthrough. They also adsorb tantalum too strongly to be suitable as substrates for the Ta-178 generator.The Bio-Rad AG1x8 system was found to be superior to the other tested systems. The effects of autoclaving, complexant additives and prolonged elution on the Ta-178 yield were measured and the chemical breakdown products quantitated.

The usefulness of generator-derived short-lived radionuclides is well established. The principal advantages are the opportunity to perform rapid repeat studies after various interventions and the use of high levels of activity without subjecting the patient to an unacceptable radiation dose. Special detectors are necessary for the detection of these high activities of radionuclides since the standard Anger-camera is not able to handle such high count rates. One is practically limited to multi-crystal cameras or gas cameras like the multi-wire proportional (MWPC) or the gas scintillation counters. This implies that the electromagnetic radiation of the radionuclide should preferably be of low energy, as these are most suitable

0097-6156/84/0241-0151$06.00/0
© 1984 American Chemical Society

for efficient detection with gas detectors. Such low-energy electromagnetic radiation can be found in the characteristic x-rays of heavy elements.

Tantalum-178 (Ta-178) is a short-lived radionuclide ($T_{1/2}$ = 9.3 min) that decays with emission of characteristic hafnium x-rays which are efficiently detected by the MWPC. The usefulness of Ta-178 lies mainly in the low patient radiation-dose per mCi injected. The high activities that can be injected generate the high photon fluxes that allow an accurate evaluation of fast physiologic processes. The principal use of Ta-178 has been in the assessment of the left ventricular ejection fraction (1,2).

A generator for the production of Ta-178 has been described earlier (1). It is based on an organic anion-exchange resin which is sensitive to radiolysis. The distribution coefficient for tungsten (W) under the separation conditions is low (2), which results in increased W-178 breakthrough after approximately 50 collections. Furthermore, the eluate has not previously been evaluated for organic resin breakdown products. This paper summarizes the results of a thorough evaluation of the existing Ta-178 generator and an evaluation of alternative adsorbents, most of them inorganic, as generator support media.

Experimental

Radionuclide Properties of Ta-178. Tantalum-178 is formed from the decay of its parent W-178 ($T_{1/2}$ = 21.7 d), and has a half-life of 9.3 minutes yielding stable Hf-178. The decay of the parent isotope (W-178) occurs entirely by electron capture to the 9.3 minute Ta-178 state, without feeding the high spin Ta-178 isomer (half-life 2.4 hrs). In Ta-178 decay, 99.2% of the disintegrations proceed by electron capture and 0.8% by positron emission. Electron capture results in a 61.2% branch to the ground state of Hf-178 and 33.7% to the first excited state at 93.1 keV. The balance, 4.3%, feeds hafnium levels between 1175 and 1772 keV. The most prominent features of the energy spectrum of this radionuclide are the hafnium characteristic x-rays with energies between 54.6 and 65.0 keV.

Materials. A number of inorganic and organic adsorbents were evaluated. All the inorganic materials are hydrates and were evaluated in combination with injectable aqueous solutions. Complexing agents were added to some eluents in order to reduce tantalum adsorption. Chelating resins, such as the pyrogallol-formaldehyde copolymer, were tested for their adsorption of tungsten. The adsorption of tantalum onto non-hydrated adsorbents such as the organic adsorbent Bio-Rad AG1x8 and silylated silica were evaluated.

The following chromatographic inorganic adsorbents were donated by Applied Research SPRL (Belgium): hydrous titanium oxide, titanium oxide-hydrogen peroxide hydrate, hydrous zirconium oxide, hydrous ferric oxide, hydrous stannic oxide, polyantimonic acid, silicic acid, hydrous chromium oxide, hydrous manganese dioxide, zirconium phosphate, tin phosphate, Phomix (20% ammonium phosphotungstate in zirconium phosphate), Siphozir (zirconium phosphate-silicate), chromium phosphate, titanium phosphate, molybdenyl ferrocyanide, zirconium ferrocyanide, ferric ferrocyanide and K-Co ferrocyanide. Alumina was obtained from Woelm (Eschwege, Germany). Tungsten carbide, non-chromatographic, was obtained from Pfaltz and Bauer (Stamford, Conn.). Tungsten disulfide was obtained from Alfa-Ventron (Danvers, Mass.). Bio-Rad AG1x4A was obtained from Bio-Rad (Richmond, Ca.). Some inorganic materials were synthesized in our laboratory. This group included tungstic acid, CaF_2 and SrF_2-coated Al_2O_3, anhydrous SnO_2, TiO_2, SiO_2, CrO_3, MnO_2, tin phosphate, zirconium phosphate, titantium phosphate, molybdenyl ferrocyanide, zirconium ferrocyanide and ferric ferrocyanide. Tungstic acid was produced by heating WO_3 with a B_2O_3 flux to 1,200^oC, cooling the melt to 800^oC at a rate of 2^oC/hour and then to room temperature. The CaF_2- or SrF_2-coated Al_2O_3 were prepared by treatment of an Al_2O_3 adsorbent, saturated with Ca^{2+} or Sr^{2+} with a NaF solution. Controlled pore glass beads (237 A mean diameter) were obtained from Electronucleonics, Inc. (Fairfield, NJ). Silane Z-6020 was obtained from Dow-Corning. Two kinds of chelate resin were synthesized and evaluated: A pyrogallol-formaldehyde copolymer (3,4) and a copolymer of alphabenzoin oxime with formaldehyde. Bio-Rad AG1x8 200-400 mesh was used as adsorbent to evaluate the published generator method (1). Silylated silicagel was prepared according to the procedure of Leyden, et al (5). Fine grains of controlled-pore glass beads (CPG) were heated for three hours with 100 ml of a 10% solution of Z-6020 silane in toluene. The filtered and toluene-washed product was dried overnight at 80^oC and used as a tungsten-adsorbent.

Determination of Partition Coefficients (K_D). The K_D values of W and Ta between the adsorbents and various mobile phases of interest were measured by batch equilibration. The first adsorbent was pre-equilibrated three times with the liquid phase, and the supernate decanted. The batch equilibration was performed using 100 mg of adsorbent and 5 grams of mobile phase, to which a W-178-Ta-178 mixture was added. The two phases were then shaken for 10 minutes by means of a Hematec Aliquot mixer.

After centrifugation, samples from each phase were analyzed for W-178 and Ta-178 using a Ge (Li) detector coupled to a Nuclear Data ND60 γ-spectrophotometer. Tantalum-178 was quantitated using its 93 keV gamma-ray. After correction for physical decay, the K_D values are calculated as the ratio of the concentrations of the element in the static and the mobile phase (2). Since the concentrations are proportional to the radioactivity level

$$K_D = \frac{\text{activity of radionuclide/g adsorbent}}{\text{activity of radionuclide/g mobile phase}}$$

where the adsorbent is always weighed as an air-dried powder. Tungsten-178 was quantitated after both fractions were allowed to decay for 90 minutes and by counting the equilibrium activity of Ta-178 associated with the W-178. The K_D-values were calculated as for tantalum.

Adsorption Studies. The inorganic adsorbents listed above were evaluated with the following non-complexing eluents: 10^{-3}N HCl, 0.1N NaOH, 0.25% $Na_2HPO_4.7H_2O$, 0.9% NaCl and 0.1% $NaHSO_3$. The adsorption of W and Ta onto organic adsorbents was also evaluated. The W and Ta adsorption onto the pyrogallol-formaldehyde resin was evaluated with aqueous mobile phases as a function of pH. The K_D of W and Ta between silica or silylated silica and mobile phases containing dilute HCl or 1% NaF were determined. An attempt to improve the adsorption of W onto Dowex 1x8 was made by converting the loaded W-178 activity to phosphotungstate, either by recrystallizing the phosphotungstate and using its HCl solutions or by forming it *in situ* by means of H_3PO_4 and direct evaluation of this solution. The K_D values for W and Ta between Bio-Rad AG1x4 and HCl solutions of differing normality were also determined. The effect of the addition of 10^{-2} M or 10^{-1} M H_3PO_4 to the 0.1 N HCl mobile phases was measured. The K_D values for W and Ta between either HCl or NaF solutions and the chelating resin Chelex 100 were determined as a function of the pH of the mobile phase.

The adsorption of W and Ta onto inorganic adsorbents from mobile phases containing fluoride was also studied. The K_D values of W and Ta between fluoride containing aqueous phases and MnO_2, Ti-phosphate, SiO_2, silylated SiO_2 and SrF_2 were determined as a function of the pH of the mobile phase. A study was made of the rate of adsorption of W and Ta onto ZrO_2 from a 0.1%

Na-oxalate solution and onto MnO_2 from 1% NaF solutions. A study of the rates of desorption of W and Ta from MnO_2 by means of 1% NaF solutions was made.

Distillation Generator. Irradiated tantalum foils were dissolved in HF + HNO_3, the solution converted to 29N HF and heated to boiling in an all-Teflon distillation apparatus. Nitrogen was used as a carrier-gas to distil (W-178) WF_6 which could be used to generate the non-volatile (Ta-178)TaF_5. This would then be isolated by vacuum manipulation of the WF_6.

Further Evaluation of the Existing Ta-178 Generator. Shielded Ta-178 generators of 2 cc bed size that can be eluted in a short time by means of vacuum aspiration were prepared in the Squibb Minitec configuration. Generators were built using Bio-Rad AG1x8 as the adsorbent. The effects of eluent acidity and hydrogen peroxide concentration, autoclaving, column bed size variation, total eluent volume used and eluent additives on the breakthrough of W-178 and the yield of Ta-178 were evaluated. The eluate was analyzed for possible organic resin-degradation products by means of gas-chromatography. In order to quantitatively evaluate the presence and magnitude of the impurity in successive elutions, twelve "cold" standard columns were loaded with Bio-Rad AG1x8 resin and subjected to a standard W-178-loading procedure, except that no W-178 was present in solution. The elutions were performed with 0.15 N HCl + 0.01% H_2O_2. At 1, 3, 11, and 38 days after preparation, three elutions of 1 ml each were collected from each column. The pH of the samples were adjusted to 12 as required for the gas chromatography procedure. Quantitation was by flame ionization after the gas chromatographic separation.

Results

The results of the K_D determinations are shown in Tables I-IV. In Table I the data for systems that strongly adsorbed both W and Ta are summarized. Table II contains data on those systems which strongly adsorb only Ta. In Table III the systems that poorly adsorbed W are described. The effect of acidity on the adsorption of W and Ta onto a pyrogallol-formaldehyde chelate resin is summarized in Table IV. The K_D values of W and Ta between silica or silylated silica and 1% NaF solutions of different pH values are summarized in Figure 1 (lines 3 and 3A). The K_D values for the same adsorbents but using different concentrations of HCl in the eluent are summarized in Table V.

Table I. K_D Values for W and Ta Between Various Eluents and Inorganic Adsorbents with a High Affinity for Both Elements

Adsorbent/ Eluent	10^{-3}N HCl	H_2O	0.1N NaOH	0.25% $PO4^{3-}$	0.9% NaCl	0.1% $NaHSO_3$
$TiO_2.H_2O_2$						
K_{DW}	>2500	>500	59	>1300	>1300	>1000
K_{DTa}	>200	>400	>140	>300	>350	>300
Fe_2O_3/K_{DW}	>2400	>1000		>125	>800	>800
K_{DTa}	>500	>250		>125	>200	>170
Sb_2O_5/K_{DW}	>250			>600	>900	>800
K_{DTa}	>100			>200	>200	>200
MnO_2/K_{DW}	2100		95	800	5600	
K_{DTa}	>350		>200	>300	>800	
Ti-phosph/						
K_{DW}	275		140	380	1100	
K_{DTa}	>150		>110	>200	>200	
Fe(111)/ ferrocy/						
K_{DW}	1500		125	470	800	
K_{DTa}	>140		>140	>90	>60	
ZrO_2/K_{DW}	>100	>400			>250	>250
K_{DTa}	>200	>100			>50	>50

Table II. K_D of Tantalum Between Various Eluents and Inorganic Adsorbents with a High Affinity for Tantalum

Absorbent/ Mobile Phase	10^{-3}N HCl	0.1N NaOH	0.25% $PO_4$3-	0.9% NaCl	0.1% $NaHSO_3$
TiO_2	>200	>30	>60	>150	>300
$SnO_2(CaCl_2)$	>200	>40	>200	>250	
Zr(ferrocy)	>250	>50			
Ni(ferrocy)	>200	>70			
Ti(ferrocy)	>300	>90			
K-Co(ferrocy)	>300	>180	>60	>70	
WS_3	>100				>100

Table III. K_D Values of W Between Various Eluents and Inorganic Adsorbents with Low Affinity for Tungsten

Adsorbent/ Mobile Phase	10^{-3}N HCl	H_2O	0.1N NaOH	0.25% $PO_4$3-	0.7% NaCl +0.2% $NaHCO_3$	0.9% NaCl	0.1% $NaHSO_3$
SnO_2	30	68	41	6	5	120	18
SiO_2	27		7			3	
Neutral Al_2O_3	30		6	8			
CrO_3	2		2	3		3	
Zr-phosph	15	44	16	89	55	96	55
Sn-phosph	4	14	8	51	28	78	35
Tungsten Carbide	5		1	36	6	12	24
Phomix		34	17				
Siphozir		53	12				
Cr-phosph	3		4				
Cu-ferrocy	8		10				
MoO_2(ferrocy)	7						
TiO_2	95	110	10	17	21		
Al_2O_3/CaF_2	3		3	6		28	
Al_2O_3/SrF_2	6		8	15		20	
WS_3			2	24	2		6

Table IV. K_D of W and Ta Between P-F Resin and HCl Solutions

- log N(HCl)	K_D, W		K_D, Ta	
	Adsorption	Desorption	Adsorption	Desorption
1	285	2,500	210	2,000
2	420	3,250	310	2,000
3	490	3,900	200	2,000
4	350	2,850	220	2,000

Table V. K_D of W and Ta Between Silica or Silylated Silica and Aqueous Dilute HCl

- log N(HCl)	K_D, W		K_D, Ta	
	Adsorption	Desorption	Adsorption	Desorption
		Silylated silica		
1	650	>5,000	>500	>500
2	19	130	>500	>100
3	28	16	>20	>10
		Silica		
1	26	450	>20	>200
2	30	850	>20	>500
3	56	>5,000	>20	>1,000

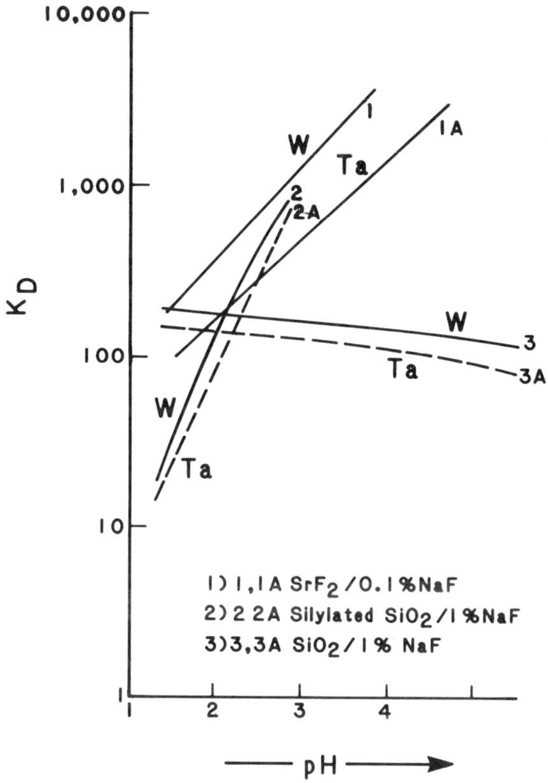

Figure 1. Distribution coefficients (K_D) of W and Ta between SrF_2, silylated SiO_2 or SiO_2 and aqueous NaF solutions as a function of the pH of the mobile phase.

The results of the adsorption experiments using Bio-Rad AG1x8 with the W-phosphotungstate were negative because stronger Ta-adsorption occurred with these phosphate-containing solutions. The results of the K_D determination for W and Ta between Bio-Rad AG1-x4 and HCl solutions of different normality are summarized in Figure 2. The effect of the addition of H_3PO_4 to the 0.1 N HCl mobile phase is also indicated. The results of the K_D determinations for W and Ta between Chelex 100 and dilute HCl solutions are shown in Table VI. The results for Chelex 100 using 1% NaF solutions of varying pH are summarized in Table VII. The K_D of W and Ta between MnO_2 and aqueous solutions of differing NaF concentrations and pH are summarized in Figure 3. The K_D values for W and Ta between Titanium phosphate and either 1% NaF or 0.1% NaF solutions as a function of pH are shown in Table VIII. The K_D values as a function of pH for W and Ta between SrF_2 and 0.1% NaF solutions are summarized in Figure 1 (lines 1 and 1A). In Figure 1 the K_D values of W and Ta between SiO_2 (lines 2 and 3A) or silylated SiO_2 (lines 2 and 2A) and 1% NaF solutions as a function of pH are summarized.

The results of the determination of the adsorption rates of W and Ta onto ZrO_2 and MnO_2 are shown in Figure 4. Lines 1 and 2 show the adsorption of W and Ta onto MnO_2 from 1% NaF solutions. Lines 3 and 4 depict the adsorption of W and Ta by ZrO_2 from a 0.1% sodium oxalate solution. Lines 5 and 6 of Figure 4 show the desorption of W and Ta from MnO_2 by 1% NaF solutions. Using the Minitec configuration, a full bolus of Ta-178 was eluted from the 2 cc Bio-Rad AG1-x8 columns by means of 1.5 ml of HCl 0.15 N + 0.01% H_2O_2. The elution is performed with an evacuated vial and takes only 15 seconds. The adsorbent bed can be left dry between elutions.

In the distillation experiment, (W-178)WF_6 could not be distilled from the 29 N HF solutions, using the all-Teflon distillation apparatus.

The elution yield for Ta-178 from Bio-Rad AG1-x8 by means of 1.5 ml of 0.10 N HCl + 0.01% H_2O_2 or 1.5 ml of 0.15 N HCl + 0.01% H_2O_2 was 33% and 52%, respectively. The Ta-178 yields and W-178 breakthrough values obtained with 2 ml of 0.15 N HCl containing variable amounts of H_2O_2 are shown in Table IX. Table X shows

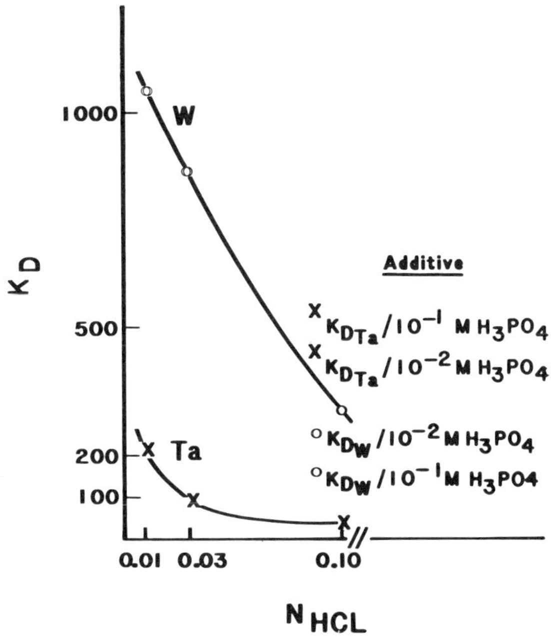

Figure 2. Distribution coefficients (K_D) of W and Ta between Bio-Rad AG1x4 and aqueous HCl solutions as a function of HCl concentration.

Table VI. K_D of W and Ta Between Chelex 100 and Mobile Phases of Varying HCl Concentration (10' Desorption)

pH	K_D W	K_D Ta
0.6	950	100
0.8	1,250	150
1.0	3,000	400
1.1	3,000	-
1.3	4,000	500
4.8	75	40
9.0	10	10
	10	20

Table VII. K_D of W and Ta Between Chelex 100 and 1% NaF Aqueous Solutions as a function of pH (10' desorption)

pH	K_D W	K_D Ta
1.8	1,600	85
2.0	300	100
3.1	350	80
3.9	-	90
5.1	130	40
6.0	170	50
7.4	30	25
8.3	20	20
8.7	10	10
9.9	1	2

Table VIII. K_D of W and Ta Between Ti-phosphate and fluoride solutions as a function of pH

pH	1% NaF K_D		pH	0.1% NaF K_D	
	W	Ta		W	Ta
0.4	42	22	1.1	230	>250
0.8	150	50	1.5	890	410
1.3	90	70	2.0	360	175
1.6	270	150	3.0	420	160
2.1	320	200	3.4	450	160
4.0	760	140	4.3	780	200
5.4	920	120	4.7	1,250	340
6.0	1,900	170	5.0	1,450	340
6.4	530	370	5.1	1,100	320
6.6	460	>500	5.2	1,100	330

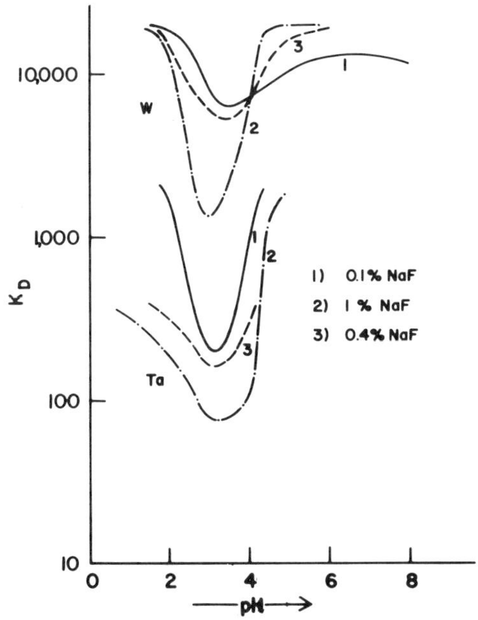

Figure 3. Distribution coefficients (K_D) of W and Ta between MnO_2 and aqueous NaF solutions of different concentration as a function of the pH of the mobile phase.

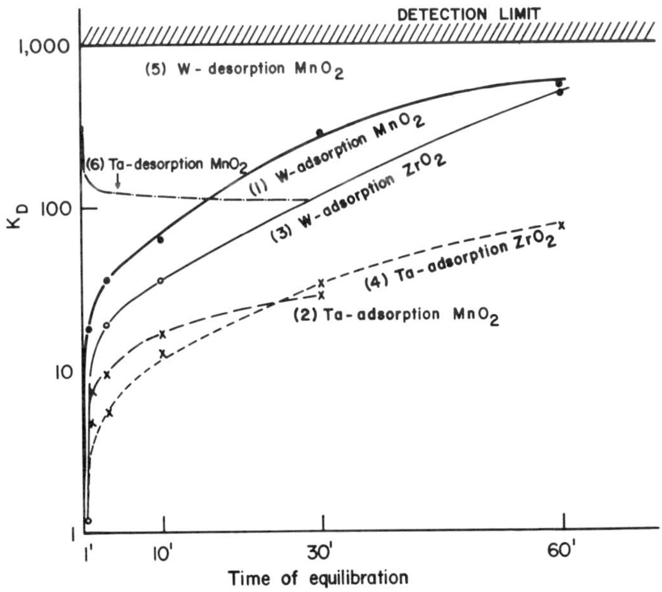

Figure 4. Adsorption rate of W and Ta onto MnO_2 and ZrO_2 from aqueous 1% NaF solutions and desorption of these elements from MnO_2.

the influence of autoclaving of the loaded AG1-x8 generator on the Ta-178 yield and radiochemical purity (RCP). To inhibit the migration of particles during the autoclaving, an intermediary filter was added 5 mm under the top filter of the column. The effect of autoclaving on the Ta-178 yield and RCP for this type of column is summarized in Table XI. The results of an exhaustive elution of a 1 cc Ta-178 generator based on Bio-Rad AG1x8 is shown in Table XII. Each elution was performed with 1 ml of HCl 0.15N + 0.01% H_2O_2. Several mixtures of 0.15 N HCl with other components were evaluated as eluents for a 2 cc Ta-178 generator. The results are summarized in Table XIII. Trimethylamine was identified as a product of the decomposition of the Bio-Rad AG1-x8 anion-exchange resin. The quantitative results obtained by gas-chromatography and FID are summarized in Table XIV.

Discussion

Using a 0.10 N HCl + 0.01% H_2O_2 as eluent, the Life Sciences Division of the National Aeronautics and Space Administration (NASA) has successfully operated a large number of Ta-178 generators based on Bio-Rad AG1x8 and has successfully tested them in human subjects (5). Ultimately, their intention is to use these for evaluation of cardiac function of astronauts in space. The only published Ta-178 generator is based on adsorption of W-178 on an organic anion-exchanger and elution of the daughter isotope by means of a dilute HCl eluent, containing a small amount of H_2O_2. The eluate can easily be converted to an injectable solution and the Ta-178 yields in 1 ml eluent volume are higher than 50%. However, the W-breakthrough increases to more than 0.1% after about 50 collections. The early breakthrough and the radiolytic instability of organic adsorbents are the main drawbacks of this system. An attempt to correct these shortcomings by using a more radiation-resistant inorganic adsorber or with any other adsorbent that would adsorb W more strongly than Bio-Rad AG1x8 did not lead to a procedure that was superior to the original system. Many inorganic adsorbents have a high affinity for tungsten but typically also adsorb tantalum very strongly. It was noted that Ta-178 which had grown in from W-178 while the latter was adsorbed was very strongly retained by all the inorganic adsorbents. The reason for this strong Ta binding may result from isoelectronic transition of the W-178 which probably does cleave any chemical bonds between the daughter isotope Ta-178 and the atoms or groups of the molecule. Since most of the experiments have been performed with WO_4^{2-}, the resultant Ta species may be expected to remain oxygenated because Ta 5d-orbitals overlap strongly with oxygen 2p-orbitals to give substantial π-bonding.

Table IX. Ta-178 Yield and W-178 Breakthrough from Bio-Rad AG1x8 as a Function of the H_2O_2-Concentration

% H_2O_2	Ta-178 Yield (%)	W-178 Breakthrough ($x10^3$)
0	17	5
0.01	48	0.2
0.05	54	N.A.
0.10	38	<0.2
0.20	55	N.A.
0.50	51	N.A.

N.A. = Not Available

Table X. Ta-178 Yield and RCP Before and After Autoclaving of the Loaded Generator

Eluent Volume (ml)	Ta-178 Yield (%)		W-178 Breakthrough	
	Before	After	Before	After
1	48 (n=5)	42	<0.1(n=5)	5(n=5)
1.5	45 (n=5)	N.A.	<0.1(n=5)	N.A.

Table XI. Effect of Autoclaving on Ta-178 Yield and RCP for the Modified Column

	Ta-178 Yield		W-178 Breakthrough ($x10^3$)	
Eluent	Before	After	Before	After
HCl 0.15N + 0.1% H_2O_2	48(n=5)	47(n=5)	0.5	0.3
HCl 0.15N + 0.01% H_2O_2	N.A.	37(n=5)	N.A.	0.5

Table XII. Ta-178 Yield and W-178 Breakthrough from a 1 cc Bio-Rad AG1x8 Column as a Function of the Total Eluted Volume

Volume Eluted (ml)	Ta-178 Yield (%)	W-178 Breakthrough ($x10^3$)
1 - 10	40	0.07
11 - 20	37	0.05
21 - 30	49	0.05
31 - 40	46	0.24
41 - 50	72	1.7
51 - 60	67	4.6
61 - 70	47	6.1
71 - 80	44	5.1
81 - 90	54	5.0
91 -100	45	5.0

Table XIII. Effect of Eluent Additives on Ta-178 Yield from Bio-Rad AG1x8

Eluent	Ta-178 Yield (%)
HCl 0.15N + 10^{-2} N NaF	0.3
HCl 0.15N + 0.03 N HNO3	10
HCl 0.05N + 0.1% Na_3-citrate	0.6

Table XIV. Trimethylamine Concentration in Generator Eluent as a Function of Time Between Elutions

Time after Preparation (days)	Trimethylamine (ppm)		
	1st Eluate	2nd Eluate	3rd Eluate
38	9	0.9	0.2
11	3	0.3	0.2
3	3	0.2	0.02
1	2	0.3	0.03

The initial protonated species of the resultant Ta oxides can expand their coordination sphere by coordinating water molecules. Since most of the evaluated adsorbents are hydrates, this could explain the strong tantalum binding. Tantalum-complexing agents, such as fluoride, hydrogen peroxide, oxalate, citrate and tartrate, did not succeed in desorbing tantalum from the inorganic adsorbents. A good chemical separation was obtained with MnO_2 as as adsorbent and a solution of 1% NaF as an eluent. However, the solubility of the hydrated MnO_2 in these eluents makes this process pharmacologically unacceptable. Synthetic chelating resins, such as Chelex 100 and the copolymer of pyrogallol and formaldehyde, in combination with pharmacologically acceptable eluents, were unable to separate W and Ta better than Bio-Rad AG1x8.

Our more detailed study of the Ta-178 generator based on Bio-Rad AG1x8 has confirmed that higher acidity eluents result in higher yields of Ta-178. A minimum of 0.01% H_2O_2 is necessary to ensure a good (>50%) Ta-178 yield and low (<0.02%) W-178 breakthrough. We have also found that the yields and breakthrough characteristics are unaffected by autoclaving of the generator. About 50 collections of Ta-178 can be made from a 1 cc-bed-size column before the W-breakthrough becomes larger than 0.1%. Addition of complexants such as fluoride , ascorbate or citrate has a negative effect on Ta-178 yield. The generators can be stored dry between elutions without any effect on yield or breakthrough. The only organic breakdown product that can be detected in the generator eluent is trimethylamine. We have also shown that the resin-breakdown was caused by the acidic eluent rather than by radiolysis. The contaminant increases in concentration with the duration of the exposure to the eluent but is almost quantitatively removed by the first elution. The highest levels observed were 9 ppm trimethylamine after 6 weeks of exposing the generator to the acid without any elution being performed. After one elution, the concentration drops to 1 ppm. The problem is effectively eliminated by dry-storage of the generator between elutions.

Literature Cited

1. Neirinckx, R. D.; Jones, A. G.; Davis, M. A.; Harris, G. I.; Holman, B.L. J. Nucl. Med. 1978, 19, 514-519.
2. Neirinckx, R. D.; Davis, M. A.; Holman, B. L. Int. J. Appl. Radiat. Isot. 1981, 32, 85-89.
3. Neirinckx, R. D.; Davis, M. A. J. Nucl. Med. 1979, 20, 681.
4. Neirinckx, R. D.; Davis, M. A. In "Radiopharmaceutical II"; Society of Nuclear Medicine: New York, N.Y. 1979; pp. 791-799.
5. Babich, J. W., personal communication.

RECEIVED October 5, 1983

11

Electrochemistry as a Basis for Radiochemical Generator Systems

G. E. BENTLEY, F. J. STEINKRUGER, and P. M. WANEK

Group INC-3, Los Alamos National Laboratory, Los Alamos, NM 87545

Ion exchange and solvent extraction techniques have been used extensively as the basis for radiochemical generators exploiting the differences in absorption behavior between the parent nuclide and its useful daughter nuclide. Many parent/daughter pairs of nuclides have sufficiently different polarographic half wave potentials so that their electrochemical behavior may be exploited for rapid separation of the daughter from the parent with minimal contamination of the product with the parent isotope.

Radionuclide generators provide a convenient method by which short-lived radioisotopes may be used without the problems associated with onsite production of short-lived materials. Generators utilize a relatively long-lived parent isotope from which the desired daughter isotope may be readily separated. Chemical methods that have been extensively exploited for the separation of daughter from parent isotopes have included adsorption column, solvent extraction and volatility methods (1). Examples of generators for short-lived nuclides include the familiar Mo-99/Tc-99m alumina column system which is the most widely used because of the desirable decay characteristics of Tc-99m, the versatile physiological properties of technetium complexes and ready availability of the generator from commercial sources. Other examples of generators that are based on column techniques include the alumina and tin oxide columns that have been developed for the Sr-82/Rb-82 and ionic Ga-68 generator systems (2-4). An example of a solvent extraction system is the Hf-172/Lu-172 generator developed by Grant et al. (5). Generators that have been based on volatility methods have not gained significant use because of poor recovery of either the daughter or parent nuclide or as a result of inconvenience of operation.

The requirements for a successful nuclear medicine radionuclide generator system include high selectivity between the daugh-

0097-6156/84/0241-0169$06.00/0
© 1984 American Chemical Society

ter and the parent nuclides so that the desired short-lived isotope is not contaminated by the relatively long-lived parent. In addition, the daughter isotope should be in a form such that it is ready to use without extensive additional chemical manipulation. A generator system must also be convenient to use (1). These requirements have resulted in the wide use of column type generators because the requirements of high selectivity and ease of use are readily attained for many parent/daughter combinations. Table I lists a variety of potential parent/daughter generator systems for which column, volatility or solvent extraction generators have not been reported.

This paper is directed at illustrating the feasibility of exploiting differences in the electrochemistry of parent/daughter nuclide pairs to produce useful generator systems. The decay of a parent nuclide to its daughter involves a move from one row of the periodic table to an adjacent row. Frequently, there are drastic differences in the electrochemical nature of adjacent rows of the periodic table. Examples of such differences are shown in Table II. In each of the listed cases, the elements may be separated from one another by careful control of a potential applied to a suitable electrode.

Table I. Examples of Parent/Daughter Nuclide Pairs For Which Suitable Generators Have Not Been Developed

Parent (Half-Life)	Daughter (Half-Life)
^{77}Br (57 h)	^{77m}Se (17.4 s)
^{72}Se (8.5 d)	^{72}As (26 h)
^{109}Cd (453 d)	^{109m}Ag (39.6 s)

Modern polarographic apparatus utilizes a three-electrode electrochemical cell (Figure 1) which contains a working electrode, usually made of an inert metal such as platinum, gold, silver, or mercury or of graphite or glassy carbon, a reference electrode and a counter electrode which may or may not be isolated from the working electrode (7). The electrochemical cell potential is controlled by a potentiostat that applies the working voltage between the reference and working electrodes and allows electrolytic currents to flow between the working and the counter electrodes. This three-electrode arrangement permits precise control of the potential applied to the working electrode and keeps the size of the reference electrode to a minimum since the

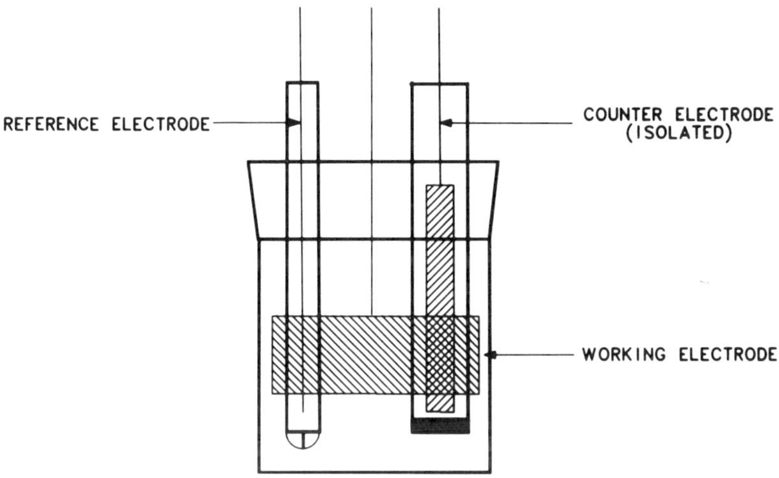

Figure 1. Typical three-electrode electrolysis cell configuration.

Table II. Examples of Polarographic Half Wave Potentials For Elements in Adjacent Rows of The Periodic Table

Species	Half Wave Potentials (6) Versus Saturated Calomel Electrode
Cd(II)	-0.65
Ag(I)	+0.05
Br^-	+0.15
Se(IV)	-0.1, -0.4
Se(IV)	-0.1, -0.4
As(III)	-0.42, -0.84
Hg(II)	+0.44
Au(III)	+0.37
Cd(II)	-0.65
In(III)	-0.71

system is not affected by polarization effects due to a passage of a current through the reference electrode. Isolation of the auxiliary electrode from the bulk of the electrolytic solution is often necessary. This prevents reactions such as oxidation or reduction of the solvent, that produce electroactive species, from interfering with the desired electrolytic reactions that are occurring at the working electrode.

The basic concept inherent in the design of an electrolytic generator system is to deposit the parent nuclide on an electrode, and allow sufficient time for the daughter nuclide to grow in. The time required for growth of the daughter is, of course, a function of the relative half-lives of the two radioisotopes. The potential of the working electrode is then changed to a value which will cause anodic oxidation or cathodic reduction of the daughter nuclide so that the daughter is stripped into the solution leaving the parent on the electrode. A second scenario can be illustrated by the Cd-109/Ag-109m parent/daughter pair. In this situation the parent cadmium is more electroactive than the silver daughter and it would be necessary to selectively plate the parent onto a suitable electrode, allow the silver to grow in, remove the cadmium from the electrode and plate it onto a second working electrode. The silver is then removed by making the first working electrode sufficiently anodic to oxidize the silver into the desired solution. The major problem with this type of generator system is the amount of time that may be required to lower the concentration of the parent nuclide in solution to a satisfactory level. It is, however, felt that this problem may be solved with suitable design of the electrolytic cell system. The preliminary experimental work that has been performed has demonstrated that it is possible to deposit radionuclides on working electrodes and to remove the deposited activity quantitatively.

Experimental

Equipment that has been utilized for scanning the useful potential ranges has included a Princeton Applied Research/EG&G Model 264 Polarographic Analyzer/Stripping Voltammeter equipped with a Princeton Applied Research/EG&G Model 303 Single Mercury Drop Electrode system. The electrode system will also accommodate inert metal and glassy carbon electrodes. A Princeton Applied Research/EG&G Model 173 Potentiostat/Galvonostat equipped with a Model 179 Digital Coulometer has been used for controlled potential deposition experiments.

To evaluate whether or not an electrolytic separation is feasible the current versus potential scans of the solvent containing microgram quantities of the elements of interest is performed using the solvent and electrode system of choice for the particular separation. The use of microgram quantities simulates tracer quantities of the elements. When the potential for either an oxidation or reduction of one of the species in solution is reached, a large increase in the current flowing between the counter and the working electrodes will be observed. The increase in the current which results from oxidation or reduction occurring in the electrolytic solution (faradaic current) is proportional to the quantity of material undergoing reaction. The potential at which this process occurs is characteristic of the reacting species. Limiting potential values that may be observed in these experiments are, in the anodic direction, oxidation of the electrode material or of the solvent and in the cathodic direction, reduction of the solvent.

Copper-67 is produced at the Los Alamos Meson Physics Facility (LAMPF) by bombarding zinc oxide with 600-800 MeV protons. A four-day irradiation of zinc oxide will result in the production of from two to six curies of Cu-67. The zinc oxide is dissolved in 6M H_2SO_4 and the Cu-67 removed from the dissolved target by reducing the copper at -0.35 volts versus a calomel electrode onto a platinum electrode. The deposition is performed for one hour after which the original zinc oxide solution is replaced with a clean 6M H_2SO_4 solution. The applied potential is changed to +0.15 volts versus the calomel electrode. This potential is sufficiently anodic to oxidize the copper that is plated onto the electrode, but not sufficiently anodic to oxidize any other species that are more noble than copper. The Cu-67 is then replated onto the electrode and the sulfuric acid solution is replaced with a dilute hydrochloric acid solution. The copper is again stripped from the electrode and an aliquot taken for Ge/Li gamma spectrometry.

Bromine is quantitatively deposited on a silver electrode at +0.16 volts versus a silver/silver chloride electrode via an anodic process involving the oxidation of the silver electrode surface (8). A 10-ml solution containing 50 μCi of bromine-77 plus milligram quantities of chloride, nitrate, and nitrite (resulting from processing of molybdenum metal for recovery of bromine-77) was placed in an electrolytic cell employing a 1-mm diameter silver wire working electrode, a silver/silver chloride reference electrode and an isolated platinum counter electrode. A +0.16 V versus Ag/AgCl potential was applied to the working electrode and the solution was stirred for a four-hour electrolysis period. During the electrolysis, a grayish-black deposit of mixed silver chloride and bromide formed on the surface of the working electrode. Following electrolysis, the solution in the electrolysis vessel was removed and counted by Ge/Li gamma spectrometry. Less than 1% of the bromine-77 originally present in the sample remained in the solution. It was not possible to quantitate the amount of bromine-77 on the electrode because the electrode presented an uncalibrated source geometry. However, gross gamma measurements with a portable survey meter indicated that all of the activity in the sample was attached to the electrode surface.

Discussion

The preliminary results from the recovery studies of Cu-67 have shown that, while the copper is not a parent in a desirable generator system, it is feasible to recover curie quantities of radionuclides using electrolytic separation methods. Copper-62 is, however, a useful short-lived positron emitter that may be removed from its generator parent, Zn-62 (9). This corresponds to the plating of a large quantity of a parent nuclide onto a working electrode. The fact that the copper may be quantitatively recovered from the electrode demonstrates that the proper choice of a stripping potential will result in recovery of daughter activity plated onto an electrode.

The experiment that involved Br-77 has shown that it is possible to quantitatively deposit via an anodic process an active material such as bromine onto a working electrode. The deposition is at a sufficiently anodic potential so that any selenium daughter formed during the decay of the bromine parent should be immediately oxidized to a soluble form. Unfortunately, because of the amount of activity available and the low branching ratio for Br-77 going to the selenium metastable state [2.3% (1)], there was only enough activity available to confirm that the bromine was plated onto the electrode with approximately one hundred percent efficiency. Further experiments will be performed when the LAMPF accelerator is in operation to ascertain whether this is a viable means to produce pure Se-77m from the Br-77 parent. Additional experiments are planned to explore other possible electrolytic generator systems such as Cd-109/Ag-109m, Fe-52/Mn-52m, Os-191/Ir-191m, Se-72/As-72, and Ge-68/Ga-68, as well as other systems that would appear to be amenable to electrolytic separation schemes. These systems will be evaluated using tracers as they become available, and quantities of stable material that simulate the tracer quantities until the radioactive materials are available.

Literature Cited

1. Lebowitz, E.; Richards, P. Sem. in Nucl. Med. 1974, 4, 257-268.
2. Neirinckx, R. D.; Kronange, J.; Gennaro, G. P.; Loberg, M.D. J. Nucl. Med. 1982, 23, 245-249.
3. Yano, Y.; Budinger, T. F.; O'Brien, H. A., Jr.; Grant, P. M.; J. Nucl. Med. 1979, 20, 961-966.
4. Horlick, P. L.; Clark, J. C.; Goodier, I. W.; Barnes, J. W.; Bentley, G. E.; Grant, P. M.; O'Brien, H. A. J. Radioanal. Chem. 1981, 64, 257-265.
5. Grant, P. M.; Daniels, R. J.; Daniels, W. J.; Bentley, G. E.; O'Brien, H. A., Jr. J. Label. Cmpd. Radiopharm. 1981, 18, 61-62 (Abst.).
6. "A Table of Selected Half-Wave Potentials for Inorganic Substances," Application Note H-1, EG&G Princeton Applied Research, Princeton, New Jersey.
7. Sawyer, D. T.; Roberts, J. L., Jr. in "Experimental Electrochemistry for Chemists"; John Wiley and Sons: New York, 1974.
8. Nydra, F.; Stulik, K.; Julakova, E. in "Electrochemical Stripping Analysis"; Ellis Horwood Limited, Chichester, Sussex, England, 1976.
9. Robinson, G. D., Jr.; Zielinski, F. W.; Lee, A. W. Int. J. Appl. Rad. Iso. 1980, 31, 111-116.

RECEIVED September 14, 1983

RADIONUCLIDE PRODUCTION AND MISCELLANEOUS APPLICATIONS

12

Production and Recovery of Large Quantities of Radionuclides for Nuclear Medicine Generator Systems

F. J. STEINKRUGER, G. E. BENTLEY, H. A. O'BRIEN, JR., M. A. OTT, F. H. SEURER, W. A. TAYLOR, and J. W. BARNES

Group INC-3, Los Alamos National Laboratory, Los Alamos, NM 87545

One of the initial concerns to be addressed when considering the development of a new radionuclide generator system is the availability of substantial quantities of the parent radioisotope. In this paper the procedures for the production and recovery of large quantities of Cd-109 from an indium metal target for the Cd-109/Ag-109m generator are described. Also, the procedures for the production and recovery of substantial quantities of Fe-52 from nickel metal targets for the Fe-52/Mn-52m generator are discussed.

The availability of ultra short-lived gamma or positron emitters from biomedical generators has been rated as a high priority item having a number of important applications. Several factors must be considered when selecting a radioisotope for a medical application. Included in these factors are the characteristics of the radioisotope itself such as emissions, half-life, chemistry and toxicity, the availability of the parent radioisotope, and the ability to achieve adequate separation of the daughter from the parent. In most cases, ideal conditions for the generator, long-lived parent, complete retention of the parent, and complete recovery of the daughter, cannot be achieved.

A generator of potential usefulness to the medical community is the Cd-109/Ag-109m system (Figure 1). Cadmium-109 with a half-life of 453 days and Ag-109m with a half-life of 39.8 seconds meet the conditions for a generator. Unfortunately, Ag-109m, which decays by isomeric transition, has a large internal conversion fraction so that the 88-keV photon yield is only 3.7% (1). Consequently, a useful generator may have to contain curie levels of the parent Cd-109.

Iron-52 has been suggested to be a useful medical radioisotope (2) and as the parent isotope (3) in the Fe-52/Mn-52m generator

0097-6156/84/0241-0179$06.00/0
© 1984 American Chemical Society

(Figure 2). In either case, the 8.28-hour half-life of Fe-52 (1) presents a problem with respect to the delivery of a significant quantity of the radioisotope to a potential user. Because of the shipping time involved, a factor of four to eight times more Fe-52 must be shipped in order to provide the user with a desired quantity. Therefore, a substantial amount of Fe-52 must be produced and recovered.

This paper addresses the availability of large quantities of Cd-109 and Fe-52 parent radioisotopes for the applications described above.

Experimental

Cadmium-109

Irradiation. Indium metal was melted into a stainless steel tube, 1.9 cm diam by 7.6 cm high, which was then welded closed. This tube was placed in a three-tube holder in an isotope production target carrier for irradiation at the Isotope Production Facility of the Los Alamos Meson Physics Facility (LAMPF) at Los Alamos National Laboratory. The target carrier, handling, and irradiation facilities have been described elsewhere (4-6). The target was exposed to 800-MeV protons for a predetermined period of time. Following proton irradiation the target was returned to the hot cell facilities of the Los Alamos Medical Radioisotope Research Group (7) where the sealed tube was cut open.

Chemistry. The indium metal was melted (mp 156°C) into a flask where it was dissolved in hot 6 M HCl. Since the target material was known to contain Sb impurity, filtration was required at this point in the procedure. After filtration the solution was adjusted to 3 M HCl by the addition of a suitable volume of distilled water. Table I is a list of the elements that must be separated to obtain pure Cd-109. This solution was applied to an AG-1X8 anion column, 200 to 400 mesh (8). The column was 1.2 cm in diameter with a total bed volume dependent on the quantity of target used. Bed volumes of 20 ml and 40 ml were successfully used.

Table I. Elements Produced by Proton Bombardment of Indium

Co	Rh
Rb	Ag
Sr	Cd
Y	In
Ru	Sn

After the target solution had passed through the column the resin was eluted with 40 void volumes of 3 M HCl to remove all the indium isotopes. The column was then rinsed with 15 void volumes of 8 M HCl to remove Rh isotopes. Cadmium-109 was recovered with 12 M HCl. A schematic diagram of the separation procedure is given in Figure 3.

Iron-52

Irradiation. Nickel metal disks, 2.5 cm in diameter by 0.16 cm thick, were used as targets for the production of Fe-52. Five disks were sandwiched with aluminum spacers and placed into a copper ring. This target assembly was placed in a target carrier and exposed to 800-MeV protons for approximately 17 hours (4-6). The target was returned to the hot cell facilities for processing (7).

Chemistry. The nickel disks were dissolved in warm 10 M HNO_3. The dissolution rate is surface area dependent, hence, the spacers were used to permit separation of the disks after irradiation. After HNO_3 dissolution the solution was taken to dryness and the residue was redissolved in 6 M HCl. Table II lists the elements that must be removed to obtain pure Fe-52.

Table II. Elements Produced by Proton Bombardment of Nickel

Be	Fe
V	Co
Cr	Ni
Mn	Cu

An oxidant, H_2O_2, was added to the HCl solution of the Ni target for valence state control. This solution was applied to an AG1-X8, 200-400 mesh anion column of 125 ml bed volume (void volume = 50 ml) (8). After the target solution had passed through the column two void volumes of 6 M HCl containing H_2O_2 were used to rinse the column. Ten void volumes of 4 M HCl, containing H_2O_2, were used to elute all the cobalt isotopes. Then the column was eluted with seven void volumes of 2.5 M HCl containing H_2O_2 to remove copper. Finally, Fe-52 was recovered with eight void volumes of 0.1 M HCl. Figure 4 is a schematic diagram of this separation procedure.

$$^{109}\mathrm{Cd} \xrightarrow[\text{E.C.}]{453\ \text{d}} {}^{109m}\mathrm{Ag} \xrightarrow[\substack{0.088\ \text{MeV} \\ (3.73\ \%)}]{39.8\ \text{s}} {}^{109}\mathrm{Ag}\ (\text{STABLE})$$

Figure 1. Ag-109m Generator

$$^{52}\mathrm{Fe} \xrightarrow[\substack{\beta^{+}(57\%) \\ .167\ \text{MeV}}]{8.3\ \text{hr}} {}^{52m}\mathrm{Mn} \xrightarrow[\substack{1.4\ \text{MeV} \\ (98\%)}]{21.1\ \text{m}} {}^{52}\mathrm{Cr}\ (\text{STABLE})$$

Figure 2. Mn-52m Generator

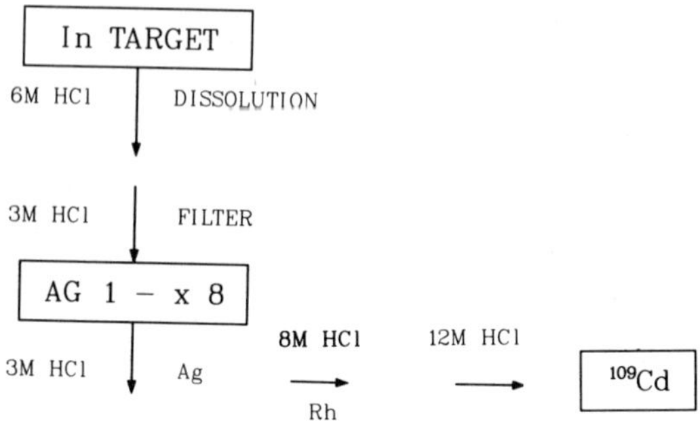

Figure 3. Cd-109 Procedure

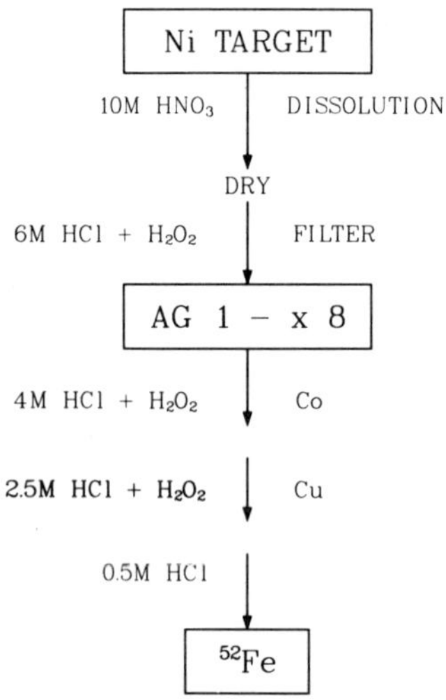

Figure 4. Fe-52 Procedure

Results

Table III is a compilation of the parameters in a typical Cd-109 production run. A sealed stainless steel tube containing 105.8 g of indium was positioned in the proton beam for 56 days. Since the beam was not on continuously for this 56-day period, the integrated exposure of the target was not available. A total of 1553 mCi of Cd-109 was produced with 1427 mCi recovered giving a 92% recovery. The only other radioisotope found was 117 mCi of Cd-115m which cannot be separated.

Table III. Cadmium-109 Production Data

Indium Target	105.8 g
Irradiation Time	55.8 d
μ•A•h	not available
Cd-109 Produced	1553 mCi
Cd-109 Recovered	1427 mCi
Percent Recovery	92%
Cd-115m Recovered	117 mCi

Table IV is a similar compilation of the parameters in an Fe-52 production run. Five nickel disks, weighing 34.7 grams were irradiated for 17.2 hours using aluminum spacers. A total of 1102 mCi of Fe-52 was produced, corrected to end of bombardment (EOB), with 1067 mCi (EOB) recovered for an overall yield of 97%. Also recovered in this procedure was 5.6 mCi of Fe-59.

Table IV. Iron-52 Production Data

Nickel Target	34.7 g
Irradiation Time	17.2 h
μ•A•h	7963.4
Fe-52 Produced	1102 mCi
Fe-52 Recovered	1067 mCi
Percent Recovery	97%
Fe-59 Recovered	5.6 mCi

Summary

Hot cell chemical procedures involving the use of anion exchange resin have been developed for the recovery of large quantities of Cd-109 and Fe-52 for use in nuclear medicine applications. Work continues on improving the speed of the two processes. Also research is underway on the development of a Cd-109/Ag-109m generator for use in nuclear medicine.

Literature Cited

1. Lederer, C.; Shirley, V. S., Eds.; TABLE OF ISOTOPES, 7th Ed.
2. Ku, T. H.; Richards, P.; Stang, L. G.; Prach, T. Proc. 2nd Intl. Symp. Radiopharm. 1979, p. 745-751.
3. Schelbert, H.; Chauncey, D.; Halpern, S.; Hagan, P.; DeLano, F.; McKegney, M. J. Nucl. Med. (Abst) 1977, 18, 642.
4. Bentley, G. E.; Barnes, J. W.; DeBusk, T. P.; Ott, M. A. Proc. 26th Conf. on Remote Systems Technology 1978, pp. 378-381.
5. Cummings, C. E.; Ogard, A. E.; Shaw, R. H. Proc. 26th Conf. on Remote Systems Technology 1978, pp. 201-206.
6. "Isotope Production Facility" in Los Alamos Meson Physics Facility Users Handbook, Los Alamos National Laboratory report MP-DO-1-UHB (Rev.) 1980, pp. 6B-7.
7. Barnes, J. W.; Bentley, G. E.; Ott, M. A.; DeBusk, T. P. Proc. 26th Conf. on Remote Systems Technology 1978, pp. 372-377.
8. Kraus, K. A.; Nelson, F. Proc. Intl. Conf. on Peaceful Uses of Atomic Energy 1956, p. 113.

RECEIVED September 14, 1983

13

The Short-Lived Radionuclide Generator

Physical Characteristics, Assessment, and Conditions for Optimal Clinical Use

M. GUILLAUME and C. BRIHAYE

Cyclotron Research Center, Liege University, Belgium

The increasing use of generator-produced short-lived radionuclides has created an urgent need for methods to quantitatively evaluate generator operating characteristics. Daughter nuclide elution yield as a function of eluant flow rate and parent breakthrough are the principal features of a generator that need to be determined without ambiguity. Standardized generator calibration methods are proposed and discussed. Clinical requirements must be considered in order to optimize the elution flow rate in relation to the total injected volume, the duration of the examination and the radiation dose to the patient. Very good agreement was obtained between theoretical values and data from experimental models using different short-lived daughter nuclides.

A radionuclide generator can be described as a parent-daughter pair from which the daughter nuclide is separated from the parent in as pure a nuclear form as possible throughout the operating life of the system. A variety of publications (1-3) have emphasized the general principles of the medical use and qualitative aspects of radionuclide generators. The most frequent example discussed is the Mo-99/Tc-99m system. Studies of short-lived radionuclide generators (4-6) do not adequately treat the quantitative problems of the daughter nuclide elution or those specific to their optimal clinical use. Two essential physical characteristics of a generator are the yield of the daughter nuclide and its radiochemical and radionuclidic purity. To realize the full potential of a short-lived radionuclide generator for medical studies requires that these two characteristics are optimized and are compatible with parameters important to clinical use such as total perfused volume and duration of the scintigraphic examination.

0097-6156/84/0241-0185$06.00/0
© 1984 American Chemical Society

Quantitative assessment of a medical generator must therefore be determined by methodologies which make possible an intercomparison of generators used in different laboratories and provide a better understanding of the physicochemical aspects involved. We have therefore pursued the development and critical analysis of reliable methods for evaluation of daughter nuclide elution yields which are generally applicable. Such absolute and reproducible methods are required for the determination of intrinsic generator parameters which determine daughter nuclide elution yield as well as parent nuclide desorption. We have also proposed a general methodology for application of clinical bolus or perfusion generators that optimizes simultaneously the activity measurement statistics in relation to the duration and the injected volume.

Short-Lived Daughter Nuclide Elution

Theoretical Considerations. For a nuclear pair, the number of daughter element nuclei (N_2) formed by the decay of parent nuclei (N_1) varies as a function of time (t) as shown in equation (1), where λ_1 and λ_2 are the respective decay

$$N_2 = \frac{\lambda_1}{\lambda_2 - \lambda_1} N_1 \left(e^{-\lambda_1 t} - e^{-\lambda_2 t}\right) \tag{1}$$

constants. When λ_2 is much greater than λ_1 and t is small compared with the half-life of the parent, relation (1) reduces to equation (2).

$$N_2 = \frac{\lambda_1}{\lambda_2} N_1 \left(1 - e^{-\lambda_2 t}\right) \tag{2}$$

In terms of radioactivity, equation (3) is used, where A_1 and

$$A_2 = A_1 \left(1 - e^{-\lambda_2 t}\right) \tag{3}$$

A_2 are the parent and daughter nuclide activities, respectively. The maximum value of A_2 is reached when the time (t) is long compared to the daughter nuclide half-life. At this time $A_2 = A_1$, if the branching ratio of the precursor is unity.

Elution Methods. For every generator, the separation of the daughter nuclide from the parent can be performed by the continuous (steady state) method or the discontinuous (bolus) method. The continuous method involves the elution of the daughter nuclide from the generator as it is formed and direct administration as a gas or liquid phase. The bolus method involves the elution at one time of the available daughter activity. Such discontinuous elutions can be performed after appropriate intervening build-up times. This method must be used when the daughter is not a short-lived radionuclide (Tc-99m). Used in this way, the generator is called a "cow system."

In Figure 1 these two methods are illustrated by the time-activity profiles measured at the output of the generator when eluted at different flow rates. The activity peak observed in the first seconds of elution is called the bolus peak. Within the limits imposed by the elution yield, this activity represents the level of the daughter in equilibrium with the parent available at the initial stage of elution. The bolus peak is followed by a constant elution value related to the rate of formation of the daughter activity. The activity eluted during this phase is determined by the size of the volume being measured. In the extreme case where a large volume is being counted, the measured elution activity is constant from the beginning and Figure 1 reduces to a single horizontal line. The value of the equilibrium level depends on the formation rate of the daughter activity (A_2). This formation rate (R) is simply the maximum value of the function, dA_2/dt when $t = 0$, as shown in equation (4). This relation shows that the maximum

$$(dA_2/dt)_{max} = A_1\lambda_2 \equiv R \ (\mu Ci/s) \tag{4}$$

level of radioactivity that can be continuously eluted from a generator will increase as the daughter nuclide half-life becomes shorter.

Table I illustrates that the theoretical maximum amount of the daughter activity that is continuously available from a 10 mCi generator is a function of the half-life of the daughter nuclide. It is clear that continuous elution is particularly

Table I. Values of R (μCi/s) for Several Common Generator Systems*

Daughter nuclide	$T_{1/2}$ (s)	R (μCi/s)
Kr-81m	13	533
Au-195m	30	226
Rb-82	78	86
Tc-99m	21600	0.32

*Values are calculated assuming a yield of 100% from the elution of a 10 mCi (A_1) generator.

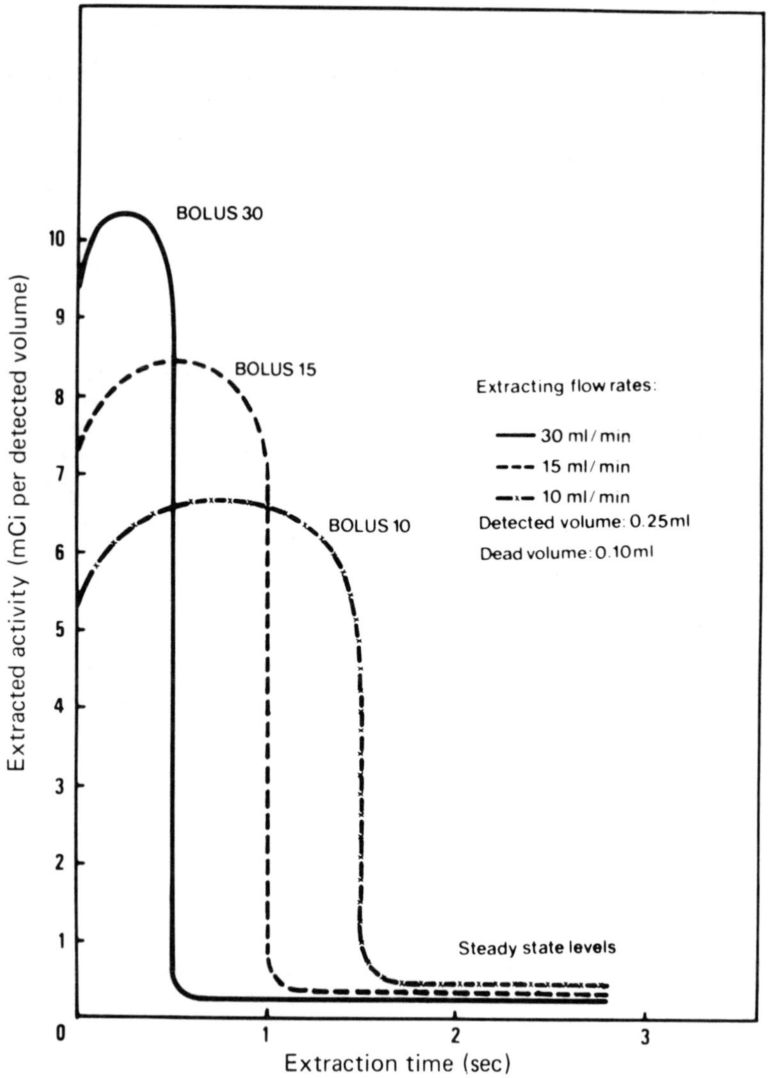

Figure 1. Time-activity profile of a 10 mCi Kr-81m perfusion generator.

suitable for short-lived radionuclide generators. In the bolus elution method when the daughter has no affinity for the exchanger, as in the case wih Kr-81m, the total daughter activity is eluted in a minimum of time corresponding to the time required to empty the free volume of the generator.

Elution Yield Measurement. The elution yield is defined as the ratio of the total eluted activity (TEA) measured under the defined experimental conditions described below to the maximum available activity, which is equivalent (taking into account the branching ratio) to the total parent activity (Q) present on the column at the time of elution. Different methods were

$$Y = \frac{(TEA)}{Q} \qquad (5)$$

studied and compared to determine the value of (TEA) in a manner compatible with the generator used and the properties of the daughter nuclide.

The indirect measurement method consists of the quantitative spectrometric measurement of the daughter photopeak, first on the column at rest and then on the column undergoing elution at different flow rates of gas or liquid. The elution yield is calculated in this case by relation (6). This

$$Y = 1 - \frac{\text{Daughter activity on column during elution}}{\text{Maximum daughter activity on column at rest}} \qquad (6)$$

particularly simple method has been adopted by a number of authors. Experience has shown, however, that this method gives experimental values that are consistantly too high, especially in the case of liquid phase elution. This method assumes that the elution yield is homogeneous at all points of the collimated area being measured and that no fixation of the eluted activity occurs on the lower portion of the column that is free of the parent activity. These ideal conditions are very rarely encountered. This method is therefore to be applied with wise reserve, and for these reasons, direct measurement methods of the daughter activity have been developed.

The direct measurement methods to determine the daughter activity proposed here involve the measurement of a sample of the eluted daughter activity (SEA) and the determination from these data the value of the (TEA). This involves solution of relationship (7) for the experimental conditions used. Two

$$(TEA) = f\ (SEA) \qquad (7)$$

different methods can be applied, either dynamic or static measurement. The experimental conditions for the dynamic method involve the spectrometic measurement of the radioactivity in a given length (l_2-l_1) of a small bore tubing or catheter from the outlet of the generator, as shown in Figure 2. In this case, the relation (7) becomes:

$$(SEA) = (TEA)\ (e^{-\lambda_2 t_1} - e^{-\lambda_2 t_2}) \tag{8}$$

with t_1 and t_2 being the entry and exit times of the activity within the measurement zone, respectively. The values of t are derived from the following relations:

$$t_1 = \frac{\pi(\frac{\emptyset}{2})^2 l_1}{D} \qquad t_2 = \frac{\pi(\frac{\emptyset}{2})^2 l_2}{D}$$

where $\emptyset$ is the inside diameter of the tubing and D the flow rate of the liquid eluant. Equation (5) can be rewritten as:

$$Y = \frac{(SEA)}{Q(e^{-\lambda_2 t_1} - e^{-\lambda_2 t_2})} \tag{9}$$

The reliability of this method becomes suspect for small diameter tubing. At high elution flow rates and small tubing diameters, laminar flow causes a very sharp velocity profile which induces an apparent change in the half-life of the moving radionuclide. It is therefore important when using this method to compare the apparent half-life of the daughter nuclide with the actual physical half-life.

The static method of daughter activity measurement can be performed in the continuous elution mode and the bolus elution mode. During the continuous steady-state elution after passage of the bolus, a one milliliter sample is collected at the column outlet during a sampling time of t_s seconds. After a waiting time of t_w seconds, the sample is counted by gamma spectrometry for 8 to 10 half-lives. Given in this case that $t_2 = t_s$ and $t_1 = 0$, the relationships (7) and (5), become (10) and (11), respectively. A typical curve of the variation of

$$(SEA) = (TEA)\ (1 - e^{-\lambda_2 t_s})\ e^{-\lambda_2 t_w} \tag{10}$$

$$Y = \frac{(SEA)}{Q(1-e^{-\lambda_2 t_s})\ e^{-\lambda_2 t_w}} \tag{11}$$

the elution yield as a function of the flow rate is shown in Figure 3 for a standard Au-195m generator.

The experimental conditions for the bolus elution mode are identical to the conditions described above except that the sample is collected from the beginning of the elution. The first milliliters contain the elutable portion of the

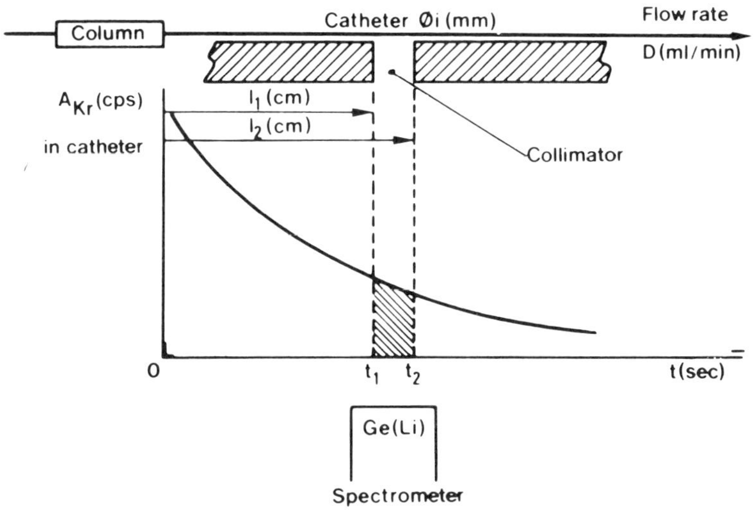

Figure 2. "Tube method" for determining radionuclide generator yield.

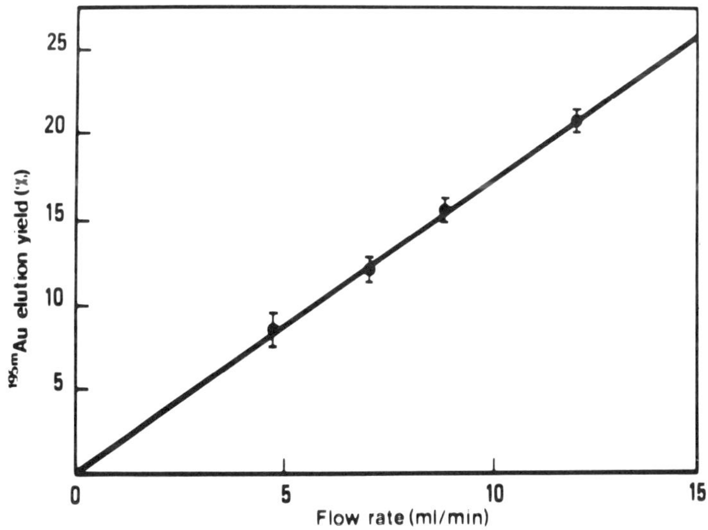

Figure 3. Typical curve of Au-195m elution yield versus elution flow rate.

activity in equilibrium with the parent and represent the maximum amount of activity per unit volume. Relation (7) becomes

$$(SEA) = (TEA)\ e^{-\lambda_2 t_w} \tag{12}$$

and the elution yield can be easily calculated as in equation (5) from relation (13). A difference between elution yields

$$Y_{bolus} = \frac{(SEA)}{Q\ e^{-\lambda_2 t_w}} \tag{13}$$

determined by the continuous and bolus methods is mainly due to a slow uptake of the daughter species by the column support. Such a comparison provides a very useful indication of the kinetics of the exchange of the daughter nuclides.

Radiochemical Purity - Breakthrough

A most important characteristic of a generator other than the elution yield of the daughter is the extent of contamination of the eluate by the parent nuclide. This contamination is defined as breakthrough which can be calculated as shown in equation (14). Breakthrough is dependent on the distribution

$$\text{Breakthrough} = \frac{\text{Parent activity eluted/elution volume}}{\text{Total parent activity on the column}} \tag{14}$$

coefficient (k_d) of the parent on the support material and on the chemical stability of the support under high radiation dose. A satisfactory distribution coefficient (k_d) leads to parent activity profiles before and then after elution with several liters of solution, as shown in Figure 4, which refers to the Rb-81 parent activity on a Dowex-50 column 15 mm in length. In such optimal conditions the breakthrough is negligible ($<10^{-6}$/ml).

Optimal Conditions for the Clinical Use of a Perfusion Generator

For the application of a continuous perfusion system, it is necessary to know what elution rate to use under steady state conditions in order to minimize either the total volume of solution to be injected or the duration of the injection. The practical objective of a scintigraphic-examination is to accumulate, in a given organ, a sufficient radioactivity to produce good counting statistics. An analytical study of this problem brings us to the formulation of the following equation:

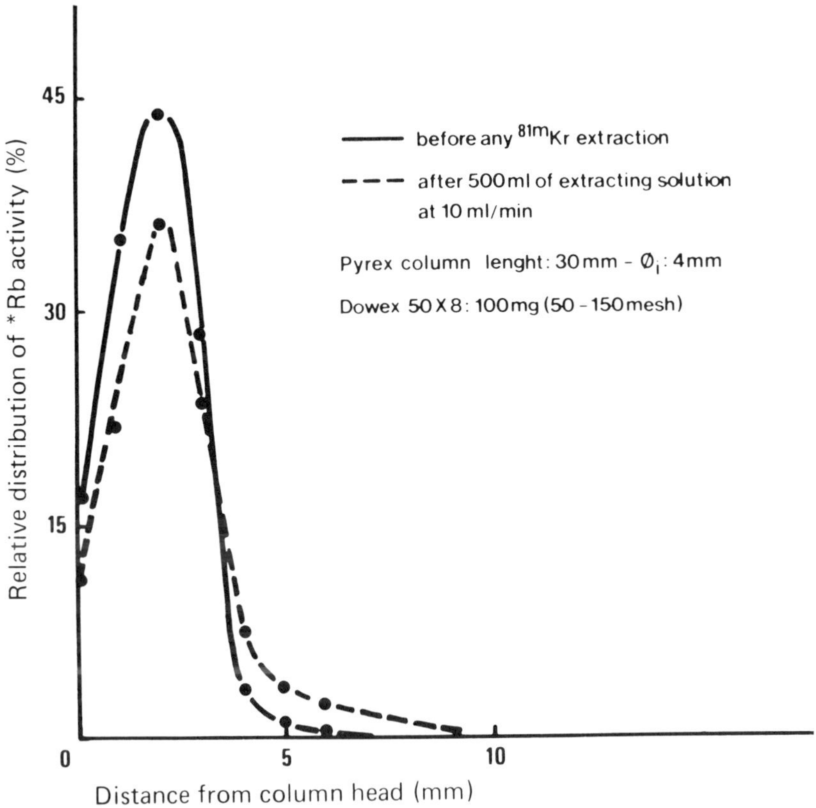

Figure 4. Distribution profile of Rb activity on a column.

$$\tilde{A} = Q \times Y(D) \times \left(t - \frac{1}{\lambda_2} + \frac{1}{\lambda_2} e^{-\lambda_2 t}\right) \qquad (15)$$

where

$\tilde{A}$ is the total cumulative activity (mCi x min) required by the scintigraphic examination.

Q is the useful parent load (mCi) on the generator.

Y (D) is a function of the flow rate D and involves the elution yield and the decay rate of the daughter in the transfer tubing.

λ_2 is the radioactive decay constant of the daughter.

t is the injection time which can be solved by equation (15).

The values of $\tilde{A}$ depend on the type and conditions of the scintigraphic examination and the required quality of the image.

The Rb-81/Kr-81m generator can be used as an example. Experience has shown that a large field of view (LFOV) gamma camera equipped with a high resolution collimator requires the cumulative activities for the three typical procedures summarized in Table II. Solving equation (15) by succesive

Table II. Cumulative Activity Values of Kr-81m Required for Typical Nuclear Medicine Procedures

Procedure	Q (mCi)	$\tilde{A}$ (mCi x min)	Counts (10^5)	Time (sec)
Pneumology	10	7.5	2.5	45
Venography	30	60	1	120
Cardiography	30	150	5	300

approximations provides the respective perfusion durations corresponding to the cumulative activity required by the medical examination. Calculating the corresponding volumes of the perfusate solution follows readily. For each type of short-lived generator, a group of monograms can be established for given activities loaded on the generator, and $\tilde{A}$, the cumulative activity required for the procedure. A typical example of these monograms is shown in Figure 5 for a Kr-81m perfusion generator (20 mCi of Rb-81) eluted continuously to accumulate a total cumulative activity of 7, 33 or 100 mCi x min during the scintigraphic examination. This example shows that the required perfusion duration time decreases very

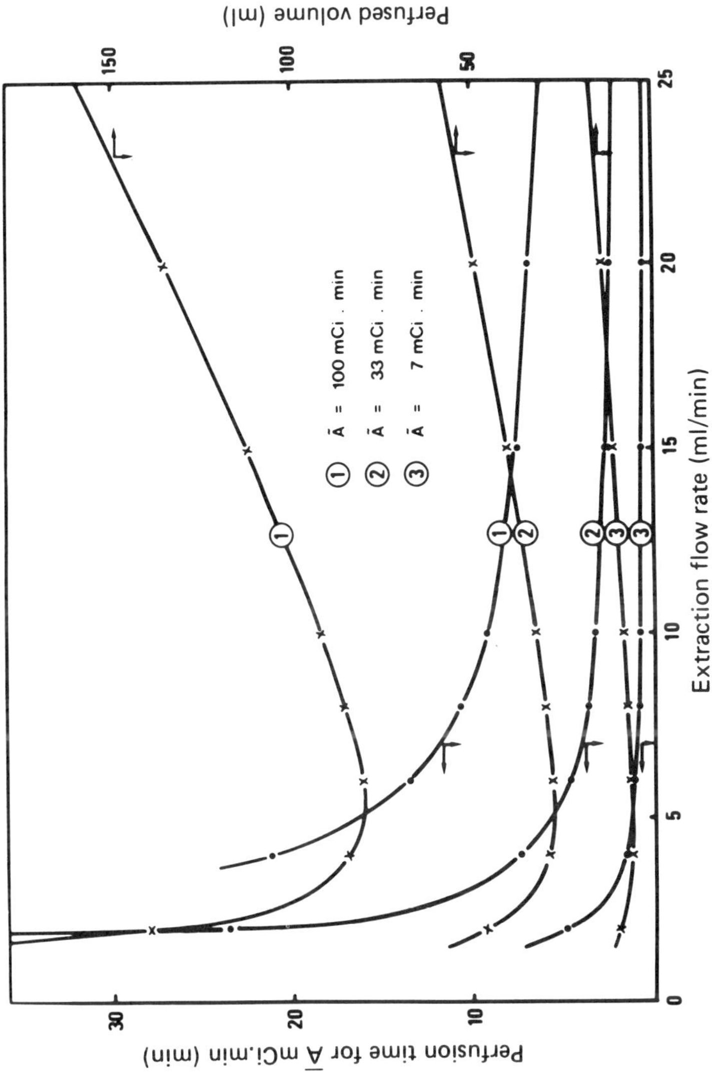

Figure 5. Duration and perfused volumes for three cumulative activities from a Kr-81m generator eluted at different flow rates.

rapidly at small elution flow rates. Above 7 to 10 ml/min, the decrease is no longer significant. Minimum injection volumes are reached between flow rates of 4 to 8 ml/min. At a flow rate of 7 ml/min, the Kr-81m elution yield is, for example, 70%. The fundamental conclusion of this study is that the optimal clinical elution flow rate in the case of continuous elution of a short-lived radionuclide from a perfusion generator does not necessarily correspond to the conditions for maximum elution yield. This conclusion was confirmed by experimental studies with various short-lived radionuclide generators such as the Hg-195m/Au-195m and Sr-82/Rb-82 systems.

Bolus Injection. The bolus mode consists of the successive perfusions of as many bolus (n) volumes as necessary to reach the cumulative activity $\tilde{A}$ required by the scintigraphic examination. A mathematical analysis of this technique results in the following equation:

$$\tilde{A} = n\, Y_{bolus}\, Q/\lambda_2 ; \text{ or } n = \tilde{A}\, \lambda_2 / Y_{bolus}\, Q \qquad (16)$$

If four half-lives ($T_{1/2}$) occur between two successive bolus elutions, the growth of daughter activity will correspond to 94% of the maximum possible per bolus and the total waiting time will be defined by equation (17).

$$t_{tot} = 4\, n\, T_{1/2} \text{ (sec)} \qquad (17)$$

The injected volume corresponding to one bolus is usually quite small, equivalent at the best to the void volume of the column. The principal advantage of the repeated bolus method is that small injection volumes are required. On the other hand, perfused activity measurements using small volumes requires high activity generators.

Summary

Different physical control procedures are proposed to calibrate short-lived radionuclide generators and to quantitatively evaluate their operating parameters. The development of isotopic generators tailored for clinical use requires that the radiochemist apply such control methods for the investigation and intercomparison of parameters of reliability and reproducibility. Clinical requirements must be taken into account in order to optimize the extraction flow rate in relation to the physical characteristics of the daughter nuclide and the requirement for good counting statistics in the imaging procedure.

Literature Cited

1. Richards, P. Proc. Symp. Oak Ridge Assoc. Univ. 1965, Chap. 10, 155, U.S.A.E.C., Inf. Serv., 1966.
2. Hnatowich, D. J. Int. J. Appl. Radiat. Iosotpes 1977, 28, 169-181.
3. Yano, Y.; Anger, H. O. J. Nucl. Med., 1968, 9, 2-6.
4. Blau, M.; Zielinski, R.; Bender, M. Nucleonics 1966, 24, 60-62.
5. Brihaye, C.; Guillaume, M.; Lavi, N.; Cogneau, M. J. Nucl. Med. 1982, 23, 1114-1120.
6. O'Brien, H., Jr.; Grant, P. M. in "Applications of Nuclear and Radiochemistry"; R. M. Lambrecht (Ed); Pergamon Press 1982, Chap. 6, 57-60.

RECEIVED August 19, 1983

14

Cryptate Complexes of Generator-Produced Isotopes

K. A. KROHN

Division of Nuclear Medicine, RC-70, University of Washington, Seattle, WA 98195

Y. YANO, T. F. BUDINGER, and B. R. MOYER

Department of Research Medicine, Donner Laboratory, University of California, Berkeley, CA 94720

We report some preliminary measurements of the potential of multicyclic polyethers (cryptands) as ligands to modify the pharmacokinetic properties of simple radioactive ions available from generators. The in vivo behavior of the complexes (cryptates) should be dominated by the highly lipophilic surface of the cryptand which surrounds the charged radioactive ion. We envision cryptate complexes with several generator-produced isotopes but initiated our measurements with longer-lived nuclides, including monovalent Ag-110m and divalent Sr-85 bound to the [2.2.2] cryptand. Murine distribution kinetics were similar for both Ag and Sr labeled [2.2.2] , giving us confidence that the ligand was dominating the biodistribution properties of these complexes. At 1-2 min the cryptate distributions were also similar to blood flow expressed as a percentage of cardiac output. There were two important differences between the labels; Sr was more stable in vivo but Ag was more lipophilic. These results suggest that generator-produced isotopes such as Rb-82 ($T\frac{1}{2}$ = 75 sec) sequestered inside cryptands may be useful freely diffusible tracers for measuring blood flow by positron emission tomography. It would be more convenient to make this measurement with generator-produced isotopes than with water from cyclotron-produced oxygen-15 ($T\frac{1}{2}$ = 122 sec).

The time course for biodistribution of a radiopharmaceutical throughout the body is a multifaceted function involving the rate of delivery of the tracer to individual tissues, the rate at which the tracer is extracted and retained by the tissues, and the rate at which the tracer is chemically processed, or for some reason egresses from the tissue. In metabolic imaging

0097-6156/84/0241-0199$06.00/0
© 1984 American Chemical Society

the goal is to interpret pharmacokinetics in terms of the second and third of these factors; yet the first factor, that of delivery of the tracer to target tissues, will always be a complicating factor in modeling metabolic radiopharmaceuticals. For this reason, physiologic tomography using positron emitting radiopharmaceuticals would benefit from independent measurements of blood flow to the target tissue. This information would allow the investigator to quantitatively separate hemodynamic factors from biochemical factors when interpreting the time course of metabolic radiotracers.

Simultaneous measurements of flow and metabolism have been achieved using simultaneous injections of cocktails containing tritium, carbon-14, iodine-125 and/or microspheres labeled with various nuclides. However, because all positron emitters involve the same gamma energy for the detected radiation, it is not useful to simultaneously inject two different positron emitting radiochemicals, one purely a marker for blood flow, the other involving metabolism. The next best experimental approach would be to make the hemodynamic measurement in the closest possible temporal proximity to injection of the biochemical tracer. This can be done best using the shortest lived radionuclides that are practical for the measurement. Radionuclide generators are the ideal source for these isotopes. Thus we are developing tracers for measurement of blood flow that are based on complexes of very short-lived nuclides available from generators.

Our initial goal was to test the potential of cyclic polyethers as modifiers of the pharmacokinetics of simple radioactive ions. Would they result in altered biodistributions that could be interpreted as representative of blood flow? Simple macrocyclic organic ligands such as cyclam (1) and the crown ethers (2) have been the subject of some investigation in the field of nuclear medicine. However, our efforts were directed toward the use of cryptands, three-dimensional crown ethers with nitrogen bridge heads (3-6). This added dimension results in an almost spherical intramolecular cavity that increases their stability for complexation with spherical cations by several orders of magnitude over planar crown ethers. Cryptands have been used in chemical synthesis as ligands to introduce cations into aprotic solvents. They are commercially available or can be synthesized easily from inexpensive starting materials and are relatively nontoxic.

Cryptates are inclusion complexes formed between cations and cryptands. Their bicyclic structure results in a flexible three dimensional configuration with a central cavity capable of accepting and complexing cations to varying degrees. Because the International Union of Pure and Applied Chemistry (IUPAC) nomenclature for these compounds is cumbersome, they are commonly described by number and identity of donor atoms in each chain between the bridgehead nitrogens. In most cases the donor atoms are oxygen in ethyl ether linkages. As an example, the cryptate in Figure 1 is referred to as M^{+}[2.2.2] because there are two oxygen atoms in each of three chains.

Cryptates are highly lipophilic molecules that readily cross biological membranes (8) and are therefore potential molecules for measuring blood flow. The in vivo behavior of cryptates would be expected to be dominated by the highly lipophilic surface of the cryptand surrounding the charged radioisotope. The biological model for these tracers might be that of an inert, freely diffusible indicator that could be interpreted by the formalism used for iodoantipyrine (9). Alternatively, these radiopharmaceuticals might be extracted very rapidly in direct proportion to blood flow, but then the cryptand and tracer might promptly dissociate within the cell and retain the ion at the location where it was initially delivered. This mechanism would lead to the experimental methods and data analysis used for microspheres (10).

Cation-cryptand complexes have a wide range of dissociation rates that correlate with the compatability in size of the cation and the crypt and with the charge on the central ion. Loosely fitting complexes are weakly bound, independent of charge. Other cations are too large and form exclusion complexes. Those of optimal dimensional matching between cation and crypt form maximally stable inclusion complexes. A compilation of literature data (11-13) has resulted in Figure 2, a plot of dissociation constant as a function of molecular dimensions. For each of the three cryptands, there is a minimum in the first-order rate constant for dissociation, representing a maximum stability.

Synthesis of Cryptate Complexes

We began this feasibility project with cryptand [2.2.2] and the monovalent Ag - 110m and divalent Sr-85 cations. These two metal ions have diameters of approximately 0.250 and 0.254 nm, respectively (14). The internal diameter of [2.2.2] has been estimated by CPK space-filling models to be 0.28 nm (3,15). Cryptate complexes form readily upon mixing a solution containing the tracer cation with a solution of cryptand. In order to insure complete complexation we used a molar ratio of ligand to ion of three. In the complexation reaction cryptand must compete with solvent molecules for the cations in solution. Thus solvents such as methanol with low dielectric constant and solvating power offer a preferrable reaction environment but we have achieved quantitative yields in water. The main problem encountered in synthesis of cryptates has been the presence of other cations such as Na^+ and K^+ competing for the cryptand. Care is taken to minimize the concentration of competing cations of size similar to the cation intended for complexation by using lithium salts for buffering solutions.

Results with Ag^+[2.2.2] in Mice. In the first series of experiments, Ag^+[2.2.2] was injected into the tail vein of restrained but alert Balb/C mice. Animals were sacrificed by decapitation

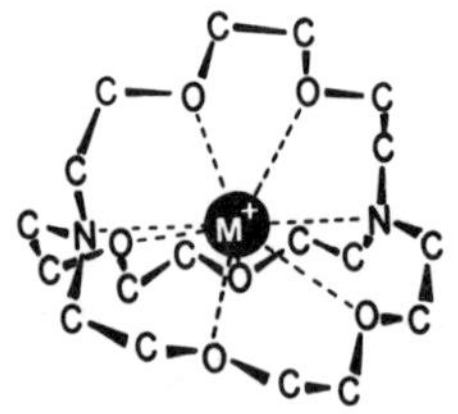

Figure 1. Three-dimensional structure of cryptand [2.2.2] complex with metal M^+. The IUPAC name for this ligand is 4,7,13,16,21,24-hexaoxa-1,10-diazabicyclo-[8.8.8] hexaxosane.

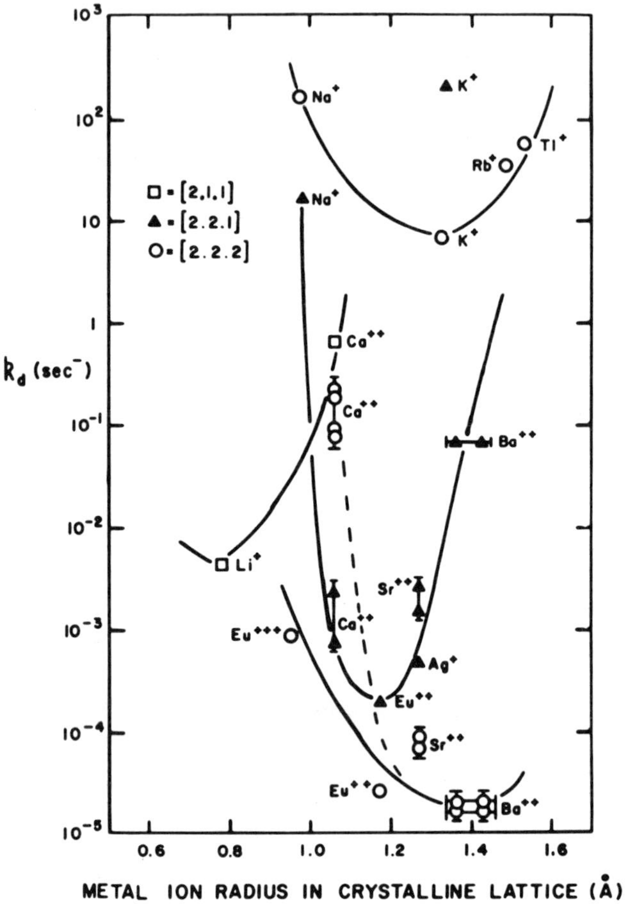

Figure 2. The dissociation constants for cryptates depend on the relative size of the metal ion and the cavity in the cryptand.

at 1, 2, 3, 15 and 60 minutes after injection. Selected tissues were dissected, weighed, counted and reported as percentages of injected dose (% ID) by comparison with a weighed standard of injectate. The resulting distribution data are shown in Figure 3. The peak concentration in all of the tissues occurred at 1 to 2 minutes after injection and correlated with blood flow expressed in terms of a percentage of cardiac output as measured by microspheres (% CO). This latter reference data comes from measurements in rats under halothane anesthesia (10) and should be viewed in light of all the precautions necessary in interpreting microsphere measurements as percentages of cardiac output. Figure 4 is a regression plot of the cardiac output data versus the maximum % ID/organ for seven tissues. The measurements for five organs (muscle, gut, heart, spleen and brain) lie very closely to the line of identity. The value for liver may be more accurate for Ag^+[2.2.2] but depressed in the microsphere measurements which used anesthetized animals and may involve shunting. The measurement for the kidney was probably more accurate by microspheres, whereas, the cryptate measurement may have been low because tracer delivered to the kidney was lost to our measurement because of its rapid excretion.

The data are also compared (Figure 3) with the 60 min distribution of gallium citrate and the 24 hr distribution of fibrinogen. These data are taken from the literature (16) and represent plasma volume to a first approximation. The cryptate distribution showed no apparent correlation with the protein distributions, as would have been expected if the cryptate had dissociated instantaneously, with subsequent tagging of plasma proteins.

The blood clearance curve of Ag^+[2.2.2] exhibited two phases when plotted semilogarithmically (Figure 5a). The initial clearance ($T\frac{1}{2}$) of Ag^+[2.2.2] was 45 sec. The dissociation reaction, Ag^+[2.2.2] $\rightarrow$ Ag^{++}[2.2.2], is a first-order kinetic process with a rate constant of 2×10^{-3} sec^{-1}, which is the stability constant for Ag^+[2.2.2] in aqueous solution at 22°C (13). Our model assumes that once a silver cryptate dissociates, the radioactive silver ion does not return to a cryptand home, but rather is bound to plasma proteins, which is a reasonable assumption. Using this model we were able to simulate the blood clearance kinetics measured in mice (Figure 5b), including the correct intercept. The Ag cryptate experiments have thus illustrated that the distribution properties in mice peaked immediately after injection with % ID/organ values that were approximately equal to literature values for % CO to those organs. In addition, these studies have shown that the activity in the brain was constant from 1-3 minutes at 0.75% ID/g, consistent with rodent cerebral blood flow (10). This implies that Ag^+[2.2.2] crosses the blood brain barrier. Also, modeling of the blood clearance curve showed that Ag^+[2.2.2] disproportionated in plasma with a rate constant equal to that which would be expected from the k_d for Ag^+[2.2.2] in

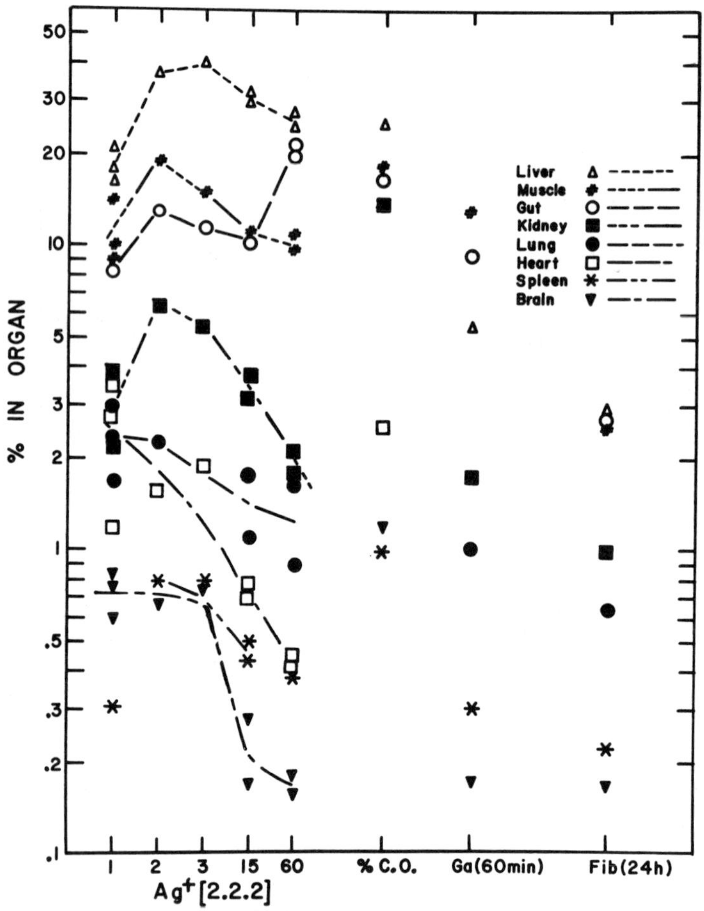

Figure 3. Tissue distribution of $Ag^{+}[2.2.2]$ in various tissues of mice. Comparison data is given for percentage of cardiac output going to each tissue and for the distribution of two common protein markers.

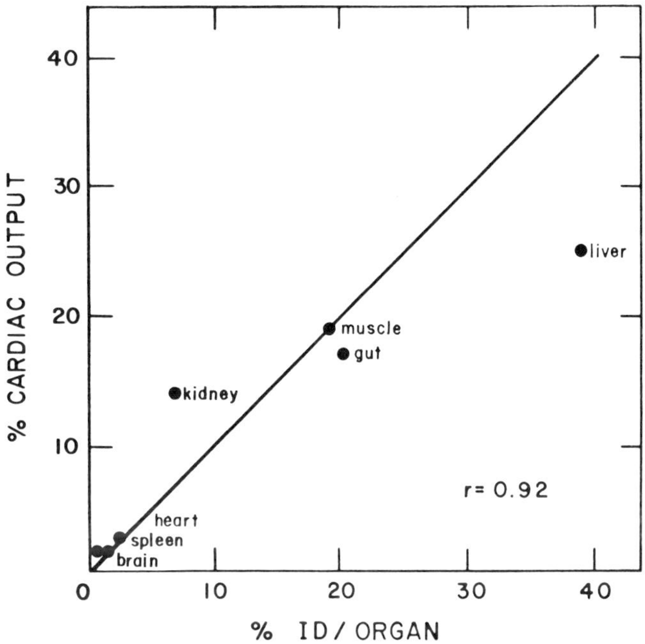

Figure 4. The percentage of Ag^{+}[2.2.2] in several organs shortly after injection correlates well with the percentage of cardiac output. The line of identity is included for reference.

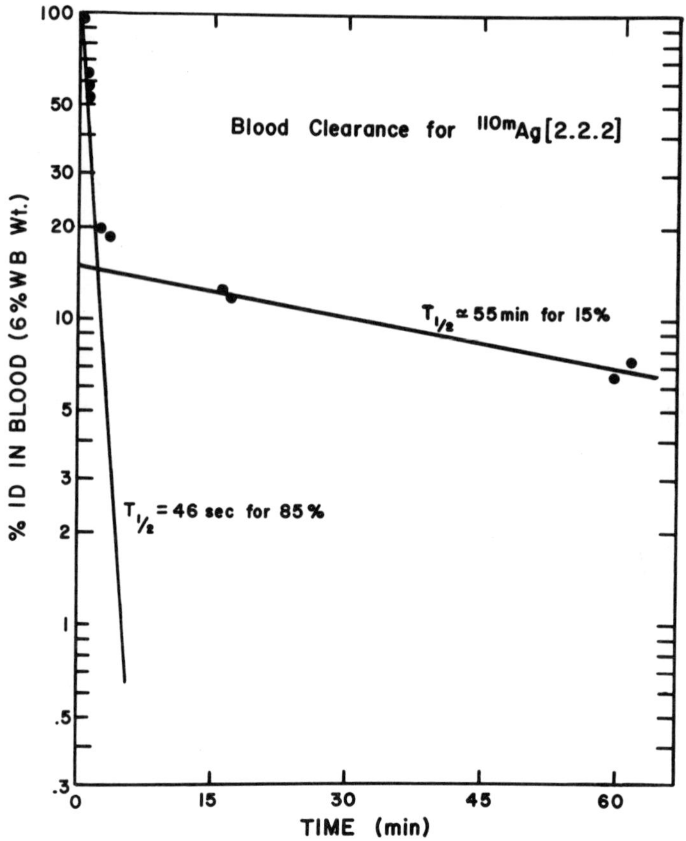

Figure 5a. The blood clearance of Ag^{+}[2.2.2] was biphasic, suggestive of decomposition of the cryptate in vivo.

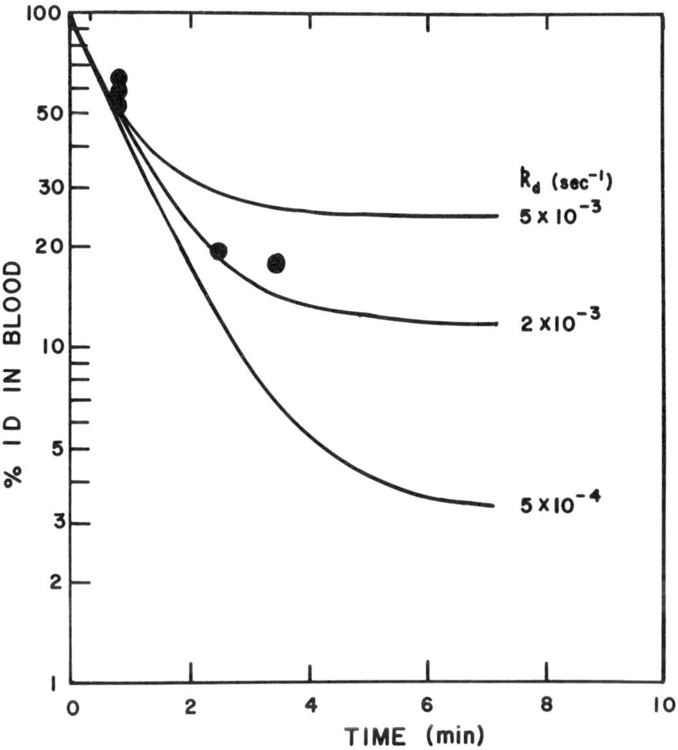

Figure 5b. The clearance curve can be simulated using a model of $Ag^+[2.2.2] \rightarrow Ag^{++}[2.2.2]$, and thus $[Ag^+] = k_d\,[Ag(2.2.2)]$. A critical test of this model is how accurately it predicts the inflection point in the clearance curve. The best fit occurred for a k_d of $2 \times 10^{-3}\,sec^{-1}$, in agreement with the literature value for k_d (cf Figure 2).

water. There was no evidence for accelerated dissociation in the intravascular space.

Results with Sr^{++}[2.2.2] in Mice. While the results with Ag cryptate were encouraging, we sought further preliminary evidence of the potential value of labeled cryptates as blood-flow radiopharmaceuticals. There were several reasons for these studies: the monovalent silver ion is very polarizable and thus may not be a general model for monovalent cations (5,17). In contrast, divalent cations form stronger inclusive cryptates than monovalent cations of the same ionic radii. On the other hand, the added charge of the divalent ion would require that the cryptand shield more charge if it is to result in an equally lipophilic complex. The above considerations led us to initiate work with Sr-85 as a tracer for cryptand [2.2.2]. Strontium-85 decays with emission of a 514 keV gamma, is commercially available and has a convenient half-life ($T_{1/2}$ = 65d). The literature value for k_d, $0.75^{-5} \times 10^{-4}$ sec^{-1}, is about 5-25 fold slower than the value for Ag^+ (13). The ionic radii of monovalent Ag and divalent Sr are equal to or slightly less than the internal diameter of the [2.2.2] cryptand.

Mouse distribution experiments were performed with Sr^{++}[2.2.2] following the protocol developed for Ag cryptate, except that measurements were done at only 1 and 15 minutes after injection. The results are shown in Figure 6 as % ID in each organ and are graphed and keyed to allow direct comparison with the Ag^+[2.2.2] data. The comparative data with $SrCl_2$ at 15 minutes are also shown. Figure 7 summarizes the limited blood clearance data for Sr^{++}[2.2.2] and $SrCl_2$.

Several additional conclusions can be made from these results. The early data for both cryptate labels were similar for muscle, kidney, lung, spleen, and gut; whereas the accumulation of Sr^{++} [2.2.2] was 3-5 fold lower than Ag^+[2.2.2] in the liver, heart, and brain. There were more differences between the results at 15 minutes since muscle and kidney concentrations were similar for both labels, but the strontium concentration was much lower in the remainder of the organs. Although the number of measurements is limited, the slopes of the organ concentrations between 1 and 15 minutes appear relatively constant for both radiopharmaceuticals and most of the organs studied. The amount in the kidneys for Sr and the gut for Ag appear different.

The control experiments with $SrCl_2$ showed a distribution that was qualitatively different from that of the cryptate. The distribution of $SrCl_2$ at 15 minutes was more like the distribution of gallium citrate at 60 minutes shown in Figure 3. These data seem to indicate that the early $SrCl_2$ distribution patterns are probably indicative of a plasma space, and that the Sr cryptate is

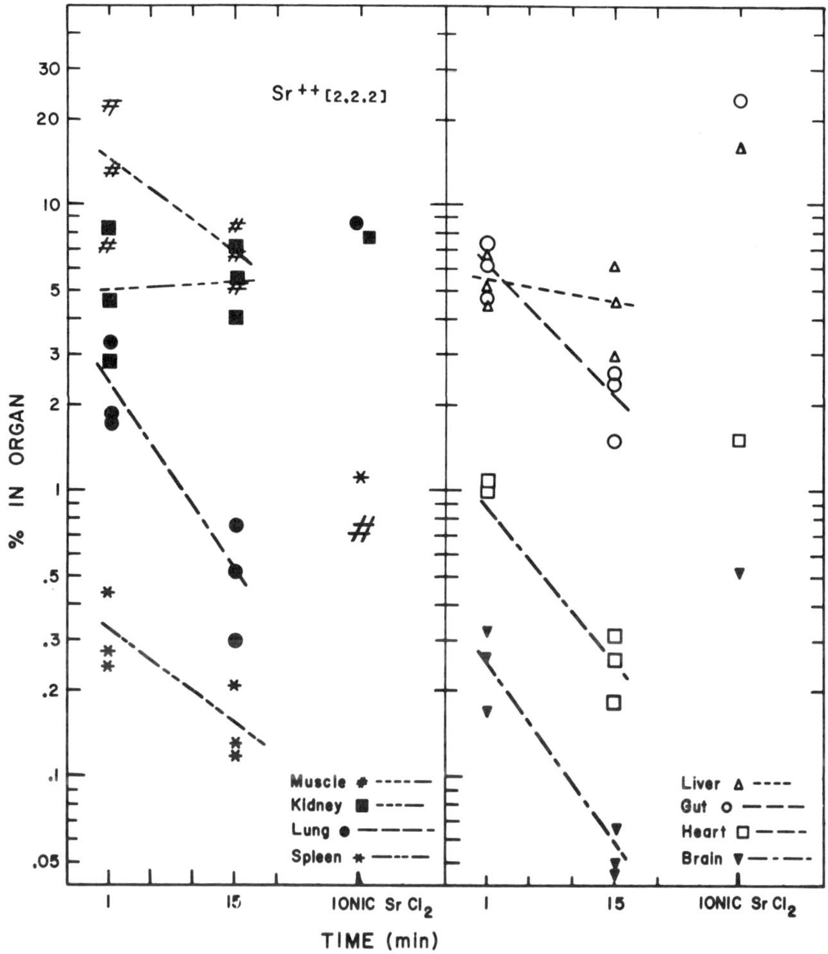

Figure 6. Tissue distribution of Sr^{++} [2.2.2] in various tissues of mice. Comparison data are given for Sr^{++} as the chloride at 15 min.

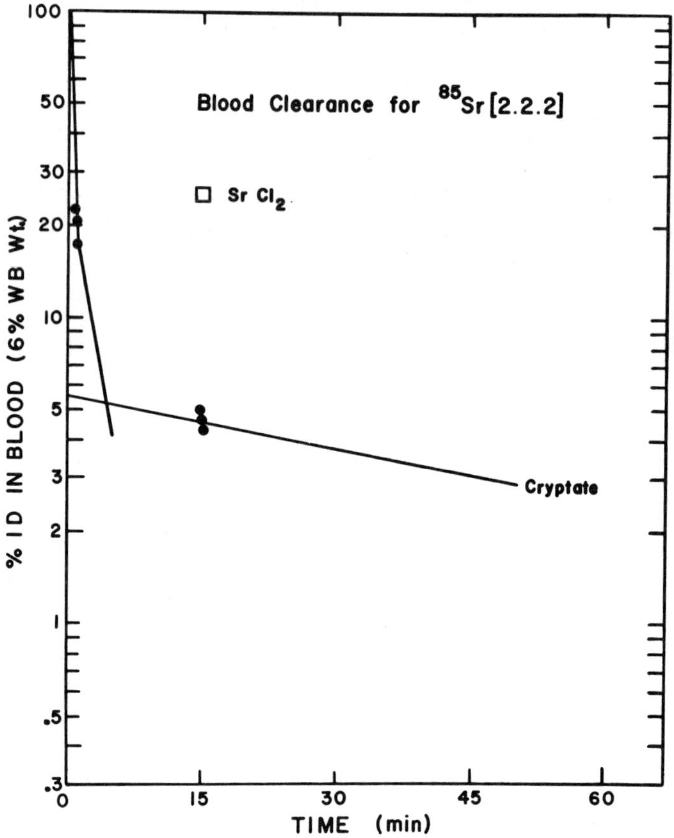

Figure 7. The blood clearance of Sr^{++}[2.2.2] was also bi-phasic but clearly exhibited a lower intercept for the slow-clearing component.

not dissociating instantaneously after injection. If this were the case, the distributions of Sr cryptate and of ionic strontium would be similar at 15 minutes.

When the organ distributions were plotted as the organ/blood ratios (graphs not shown), the differences between Ag and Sr became more apparent. The measurements for Sr^{++}[2.2.2] were much more constant with time than were the ratios for Ag^{+}[2.2.2]. This result is consistent with Sr^{++} forming a stronger complex than Ag^{+}, so that the intact complex experiences rapid exchange between the organ and vascular spaces. This property would be required for an inert and freely diffusible tracer. The blood clearance curve (Figure 7) also suggests that Sr^{++}[2.2.2] is a more stable complex than its Ag counterpart. In the case of Sr, about 95% of the tracer cleared with a fast half-life, compared with about 85% for Ag. When the blood clearance was simulated as illustrated in Figure 5b, we estimated a k_d of about 3×10^{-4} sec^{-1} for the Sr label versus 2×10^{-3} sec^{-1} for Ag.

Summary and Conclusions

The mouse distribution experiments indicated a great deal of similarity between the Ag^{+} and the Sr^{++} cryptates, giving us confidence that the cryptand ligand was influencing, if not completely dominating, the biodistribution of both radiopharmaceuticals. There were, however, distinct differences between these labels that were consistent with our predictions that the Sr^{++} label would be more stable in vivo but also less lipophilic because of its increased charge. Blood clearance measurements showed less in vivo breakdown for Sr, with subsequent labeling of the plasma space. Accumulation of tracer Sr-85 in the skeleton was insufficient to account for this difference. While these would be advantages for the Sr label, the observation that Sr^{++} [2.2.2] was not detected in the brain, heart, and liver as much as the cryptate labeled with monovalent Ag, emphasizes the problem that a Sr^{++} cryptate is sufficiently less lipophilic so that its distribution is affected by the higher charge on the central cation. These results support the potential of cryptands for making inert, freely diffusible complexes with generator-produced radionuclides. With the present data, we are unable to predict whether monovalent or divalent cations would be more advantageous labels. Other cryptands can be synthesized to give cavities with more favorable internal dimensions than those that are commercially available (4).

We envision several potential generator-produced radionuclide labels for cryptates (Table I). Fortunately, early evaluations can be performed more conveniently with longer-lived tracers that are commercially available. The cryptate complexes are conveniently formed from the metal in deionized water and the cryptand dissolved in water or methanol. The complexes form instantly upon

Table I. Generator Radionuclides for Labeling Cryptates

Isotope of Interest	Half-Life	Decay Properties: Positron % abund.	Energies—MeV: Positron	Energies—MeV: γ % abund.	Parent Isotope	Parent Half-Life	Descendent(s)	Ionic Charge	Radius A°*	Other Valence States
$^{52m}_{25}Mn$	21.1m	>50	2.63	1.43 (98)	$^{52}_{26}Fe$	8.3h	$^{52}_{25}Mn \xrightarrow{5.6d} {}^{52}_{24}Cr$ (stable)	2+	0.80P 0.93L	+3
$^{68}_{31}Ga$	68.1m	90	1.90	1.08 (3)	$^{68}_{32}Ge$	288 d	$^{68}_{30}Zn$ (stable)	3+	0.62P	+1
$^{82}_{37}Rb$	75.2s	96	3.35	0.78 (14)	$^{82}_{38}Sr$	25 d	$^{82}_{36}Kr$ (stable)	1+	1.48P 1.58L	
$^{109m}_{47}Ag$	39.8s	none (IT)	----	0.088 (3.6)	$^{109}_{48}Cd$	453 d	$^{109}_{47}Ag$ (stable)	1+	1.26P 1.27L	+2
$^{118}_{51}Sb$	3.5m	<50	2.70	1.23 (2.5)	$^{118}_{52}Fe$	6.0d	$^{118}_{50}Sn$ (stable)			
$^{128}_{55}Cs$	3.8m	61	2.89	0.44 (26)	$^{128}_{56}Ba$	2.4d	$^{128}_{54}Xe$ (stable)	1+	1.69P 1.84L	
$^{134}_{57}La$	6.7m	62	2.67	0.61 (5)	$^{134}_{58}Ce$	76 h	$^{134}_{56}Ba$ (stable)	3+	1.15P	+2

*P is ref (14), L is ref (18)

mixing and are ready for use. This chemistry is potentially compatible with generators but will place some constraints on the ionic constituents of the eluting solvent. Continuous availability of a short-lived but generator-based blood flow agent in the PET laboratory would be a welcome improvement over the current use of [O-15]-water as produced in batches with an accelerator.

Acknowledgments

This work was performed during a very enjoyable sabbatical visit (K.A.K.) at the Donner Laboratory. It was supported in part by the National Institutes of Health, HL25840.

Literature Cited

1. Troutner, D.E.; Simon, J.; Ketring, A.R.; Volkert, W.; Holmes, R.A.; J. Nucl. Med. 1980, 21, 443-448.
2. Irie, T.; Fukushi, K.; Ido, T.; Nozaki, T.; Kasida, Y.; Int. J. Appl. Radiat. Isot. 1982, 33, 1449-1452.
3. Lehn, J.M.; Struct. Bonding (Berlin), 1973, 16, 1-69.
4. "Coordination Chemistry of Macrocyclic Compounds"; Melson, G.A., Ed.; Plenum: New York, 1979.
5. Izatt, R.M.; Lamb, J.D.; Eatough, D.J.; Christensen, J.J.; Rytting, J.H.; in "Drug Design"; Ariens, E.J., Ed.; Academic: New York, 1979; Chap. 7.
6. Cram, D.J.; Science, 1983, 219, 1177-1183.
7. Pederson, C.J.; J. Am. Chem. Soc. 1976, 89, 7017-7036.
8. Pressman, B.C.; Ann. Rev. Biochem. 1976, 45, 501-530.
9. Sakurada, O.; Kennedy, C.; Jehle, J.; Brown, J.D.; Carbin, G.L.; Sokoloff, L.; Am. J. Physiol. 1978, 234, H59-66.
10. Neutze, J.M.; Wyler, F.; Rudolph, A.M.; Am. J. Physiol. 1968, 215, 486-495.
11. Cox, B.G.; Schneider, H.; J. Am. Chem. Soc. 1977, 99, 2809-2811.
12. Loyola, V.M.; Pizer, R.; Wilkins, R.G.; J. Am. Chem. Soc. 1977, 99, 7185-7188.
13. Lamb, J.D.; Izatt, R.M.; Christensen, J.J.; Eatough, B.J.; in "Coordination Chemistry of Macrocyclic Compounds", Melson, G.A., Ed.; Plenum: New York, 1979, Chap. 3.
14. Pauling, L. "The Nature of the Chemical Bond and the Structure of Molecules and Crystals"; Cornell University Press: Ithaca, 1960; Chap. 7.
15. Lehn, J.M.; Savage, J.P.; J. Am. Chem. Soc. 1975, 97, 6700-6707.
16. DeNardo, G.L.; Krohn, K.A.; DeNardo, S.J.; Cancer 1977, 40, 2923-2929.
17. Pearson, R.G.; J. Chem. Educ. 1968, 45, 581-587; 643-648.
18. Ladd, M.F.C.; Theor. Chem. Acta 1968, 12, 333-336.

RECEIVED September 2, 1983

15

Generator-Produced Bi-212

Chelated to Chemically Modified Monoclonal Antibody for Use in Radiotherapy

OTTO A. GANSOW—Inorganic and Radioimmune Chemistry Section, Radiation Oncology Branch, Division of Cancer Treatment, National Cancer Institute and Laboratory of Chemical Physics, National Institute of Arthritis, Diabetes, Digestive, and Kidney Diseases, National Institutes of Health, Bethesda, MD 20205

ROBERT W. ATCHER and DANIEL C. LINK—Inorganic and Radioimmune Chemistry Section, Radiation Oncology Branch, Division of Cancer Treatment, National Cancer Institute, National Institutes of Health, Bethesda, MD 20205

ARNOLD M. FRIEDMAN and ROBERT H. SEEVERS—Chemistry Division, Argonne National Laboratory, Argonne, IL 60439

WENDIE ANDERSON, DAVID A. SCHEINBERG, and METTE STRAND—Department of Pharmacology and Experimental Therapeutics, Johns Hopkins University School of Medicine, Baltimore, MD 21205

It has been demonstrated that monoclonal antibodies may be chemically modified by reaction with metal chelates without loss of antibody activity or specificity. A radionuclide generator has been made to provide a source for Bi-212 to be used for attachment of bismuth chelates to antibody. Such antibody-metal-chelate conjugates appear to be stable *in vivo* and may provide a new method for radiotherapy.

The development (1) of monoclonal antibodies with very high specificity for malignant cells suggests that these agents might might serve as targeting vehicles for transport of tracers or cytotoxic agents to tumors for use in diagnosis or therapy (2). Recently Scheinberg, Strand, and Gansow demonstrated that radioactive metal chelates could be covalently linked to monoclonal antibody without compromising the activity or specificity of the protein (3,4). Rapid, tumor specific uptake was demonstrated by high resolution gamma camera images of mouse erythroid tumors obtained by using leukemia cell specific monoclonal antibodies labeled with indium-111 chelates. Radioiodinated antibodies have also been employed for *in vivo* studies of protein localization, diagnostic imaging, and tumor therapy (2,5). However, the covalent attachment of iodine to tyrosine residues present in the antibody frequently compromises the specificity and activity of the immunoprotein. Moreover, degradation of carbon-iodine bonds to free iodine *in vivo* is well known (6). Therapeutic protocols would not be optimal because iodine-131 can deliver only low

0097–6156/84/0241–0215$06.00/0
© 1984 American Chemical Society

linear energy transfer (LET) β radiation as well as undesirable gamma emissions. Monoclonal antibodies localize on the cellular level and are ideal carriers for high LET radiation α emitters. Astatine-211 has a seven hour half-life, emits α particles and has been proposed as a useful radiotherapeutic agent (7-9). Astatine is a halogen and will directly react with tyrosine residues and will be subject to the same *in vivo* limitations as iodine including thyroid uptake. In addition, any astatine isotope must be produced by α particle bombardment of bismuth in a cyclotron which imposes severe constraints on the general availability of this radionuclide.

Linking metal chelates to antibodies provides a more versatile method for labeling antibodies with radionuclides. There are numerous metallic radionuclides available for use in diagnosis and therapy which form complexes stable *in vivo*. For example, In-111 is a pure γ emitter ideal for conventional imaging. Isotopes of scandium, gallium, copper, palladium or rhenium would provide sources for low LET beta radiation. The primary focus of our current tumor therapy research makes use of Bi-212 a one hour half-life, α emitting radionuclide conveniently obtained from an easily used generator, thus avoiding the problems of cyclotron production.

A Radionuclidic Generator for Lead-212 and Bismuth-212

Several years ago Zucchini and Friedman developed a long lived generator for Pb-212 and Bi-212 which was based on the decay of Th-228 (10). In Figure 1 we show the decay scheme for Th-228 and daughters. The separation of the Pb-212 and Bi-212 radionuclides from Th-228 is based upon the elution of Rn-220 in the generator. Figure 2 is a schematic illustration of the original generator. The Rn-220 is eluted from the Th-228 and Ra-224 by pure water and decays to Pb-212 which is bound by the cation exchange column, and the Pb-212 and Bi-212 equilibrium mixture is eluted from the cation exchange column with 2 N HCl. Alternatively, the cation exchange column is followed by a bed of anion exchange resin which absorbs Pb and Bi in 2 N HCl. The Pb-212 is then eluted with water (Figure 3). The overall yield is consistently between 80 and 90 percent. When the final bed of anion exchange resin is used there was no observed breakthrough of Th-228 above the 10 ppm limits of detection. It should be noted that these generators have a unique potential as therapeutic tools since 1 millicurie of Pb-212 and daughters will yield an integrated dose of 232,000 rads of high LET radiation and 25,000 rads of low LET radiation if confined to one ml of tissue.

The generator was initially used to provide Pb-212 to make radioactive liposomes for immune suppression (11). The objective of these studies was to suppress the immune response prior to organ transplant. The first studies were performed with lead-212 in nonantigenic liposomes in rats in order to measure nonspecific

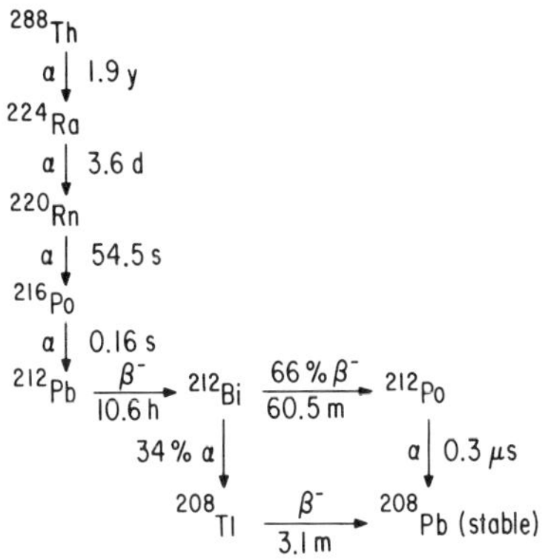

Figure 1. Th-228 decay chain.

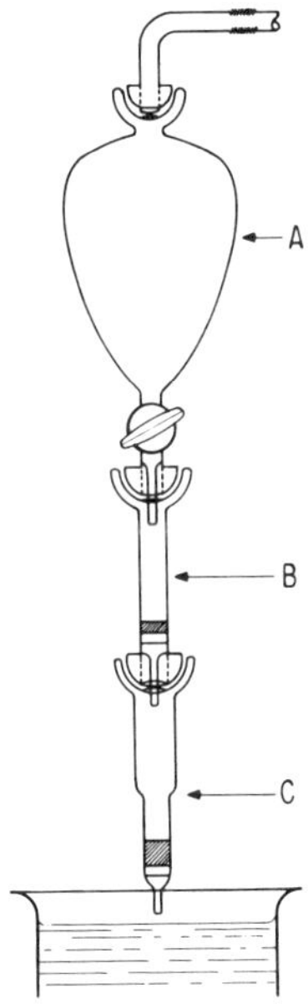

Figure 2. Generator, A = water reservoir B = sodium titanate column containing Th-228 C = cation exchange column and Pb-212.

destruction of antibody producing B cells. One day following injection of the liposomes, the animals were challenged with a series of antigens and 5 days later they were assayed for antibody production, and the number of surviving B cells in the spleen was determined. Figures 4 (11) demonstrates that the non-specific reduction of immune response correlates well with the destruction of all B lymphocytes. More recent experiments have indicated similar results obtained with phagocytic cells labelled with Pb-212 (12). In both cases it was found that about 10 decays of Pb-212 and daughters would destroy a B cell.

The generators used for these experiments employ Dowex® 1 and Dowex® 50 ion exchange resins in the elution columns. Thorium-containing titanate columns have been used for 3 yrs and proven reliable, but there has been a general breakdown of the titanate ion exchange material, probably due to radiation damage, which causes clogging and a decrease in flow rate. In order to compensate for these problems we have increased the elution pressure to about 25 lbs. At that point, usually after 6-9 months, we have disassembled the generators, repurified the Th-228, and reconstituted new generators. One additional complication has been the need for a safe facility, such as a glove box, for handling the Th-228 generator. Though a glove box has been installed at several installations, it is inconvenient and presents a potential hazard. In order to ameliorate these conditions we have recently designed and tested the new, disposble generator, based on the Ra-224 daughter (13) outlined schematically in Figure 5. We have also incorporated a set of valves to allow repeated collection of the Pb-212 and Bi-212 without unsealing the generator. This new design has eliminated the need for a glove box. In addition, the Ra-224 generators have a useful life of a few weeks and do not require refabrication. We are now developing an automated system to allow purification of large amounts of Ra-224 at periodic intervals which will allow the construction of a number of generators for collaborative programs.

The Chemical Modification of Antibody with Metal Chelates

The chemical modification of antibody by metal chelates may be viewed as requiring two distinct but permutable chemical procedures which include the attachment of a coordinating ligand to antibody and the formation of the kinetically inert metal complex. Three classes of possibly useful ligands are shown in Figure 6. The substituted cryptates recently described by Gansow and co-workers are the most complicated to prepare chemically, but could potentially carry the most lethal isotopes, the fissionable actinides (14,15). Bifunctional ethylenediaminetetraacetic acid (EDTA) and diethylenetriaminepentaacetic acid (DTPA) derivatives (16-19) are more easily synthesized and allow targeting of more tractable isotopes of the group IIIA, VA or transition metals as higher valence ions (3,4).

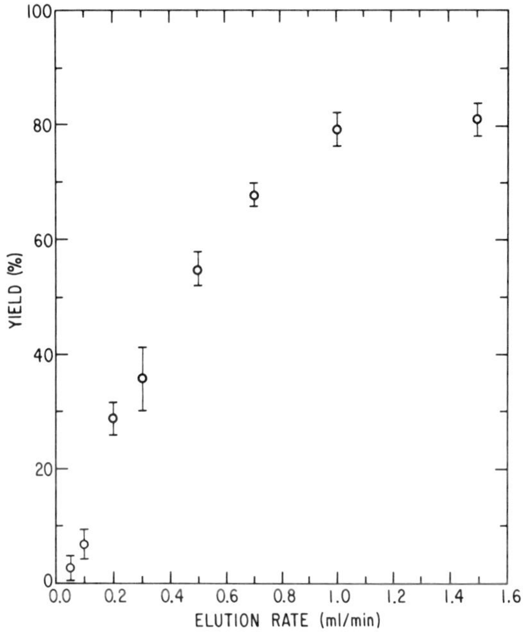

Figure 3. Yield of Pb-212 as function of water flow.

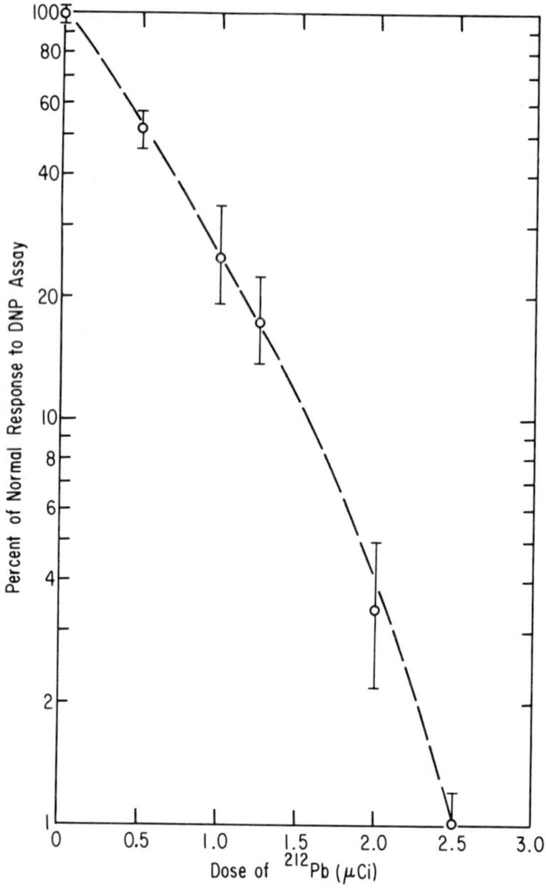

Figure 4. Reduction of immune response by Pb-212 liposomes.

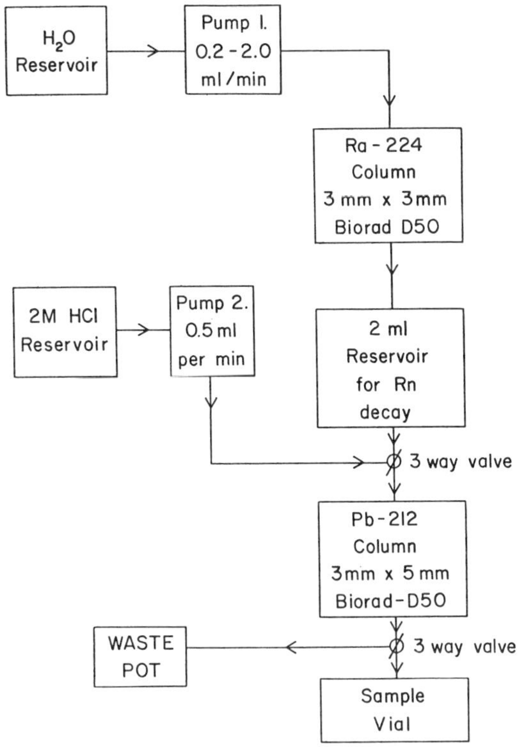

Figure 5. Schematic diagram for the Ra-224 generator.

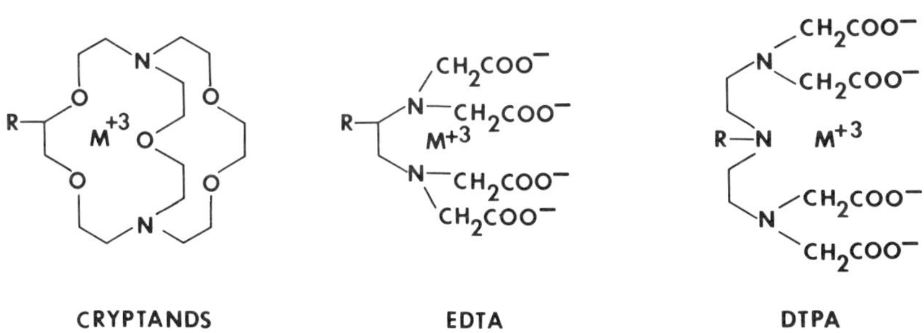

Figure 6. Three bifunctional metal chelates: substituted cryptand, bifunctional EDTA, and DTPA.

Metallic radionuclides with suitable characteristics for diagnostic nuclear medicine that can be chelated tightly include the positron emitting gallium-68, and gamma emitting radionuclides such as technecium-99m (20) and indium-111. These radionuclides all have short half-lives that vary from about one hour to three days. Isotopes which might have therapeutic effects include several beta emitting radionuclides of scandium or rhenium and the alpha emitting radionuclides bismuth-212 or actinium-225. The higher valence ions of each of these elements bind to EDTA of DTPA with pK values >24 (21). Our studies have therefore focused on conjugation of these ligands to antibody.

Chemical modification of proteins must occur at a reactive functional group on the molecular backbone. Three useful chemical substituents include the phenolic side chain of tyrosine, the ε amino group of lysine and the cysteine sulfhydryl groups. We eliminated sulfhydryl attachment as a candidate because of the well known instability of disulfide linkages in aqueous media, although if a thioether linkage could be formed, it might be useful. Attempts to link ligand to tyrosine by reaction of 1-(p-benzyldiazonium)EDTA (3,4) with antibody produced only conjugates which had immunoreactivity and specificity severely compromised. Similarly, conjugates of the p-hydroxybenzimidate of 1-(*p*-benzyldiazonium)EDTA (18) met the same fate, presumably because of the high solution pH and salt concentration required for for efficient reaction.

The first successful conjugation of chelate to antibody was reported by Scheinberg, Strand and Gansow in 1981 (3,4). A modification of the method of Yeh, et al (16-19) was employed to prepare 1-(p-carboxymethoxybenzyl)EDTA and its iron(III) complex formed by air oxidation of ferrous sulfate in aqueous solutions of the ligand. Coupling through the carboxylate to form and acid amide linkage with ε amino groups of antibody lysines was effected by the water soluble 1,3-(3-dimethylaminopropyl)carbodiimide. By use of iron-59 tracer, it was determined that approximately 0.9 chelates were bound to immunoprotein. Iron was subsequently removed by dialysis against a buffered solution of ascorbate, leaving the EDTA portion of the molecule free to be reacted with another metal ion. Antibody-chelate-metal conjugates were formed with indium, gallium, and scandium by reaction of the appropriate trivalent ion. No loss of antibody activity or specificity was measured by cell binding study. In more recent experiments, two derivatives of DTPA have proven to be the simplest to prepare and most widely useful conjugating ligands. Both the carboxycarbonic anhydride of DTPA (17) and the DTPA dianhydride (16,19,22-25) react easily with antibody near neutral solution pH values to give conjugates with no loss of immunoreactivity or cell binding specificity and are useful for imaging, Figure 7. We therefore have studied their reaction with an easily obtained immunoprotein, bovine IgG. The results of pH and concentration dependence of ligand-protein conjugation are shown in Figures 8-10. In general, efficiency of conjugation is

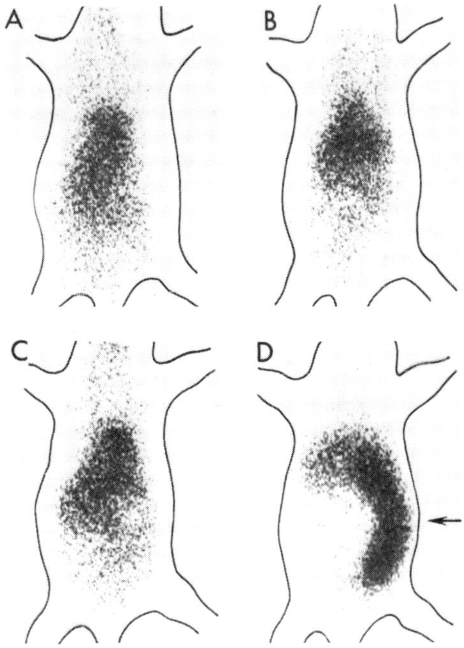

Figure 7. Images of normal and leukemic mice injected with In-111 DTPA-labeled monoclonal antibodies. A,B (normal) and C,D (leukemic) were injected with control (A,C) or tumor-specific (B,D) antibody. Reproduced with permission from Ref. 4. Copyright 1982, American Association for the Advancement of Science.

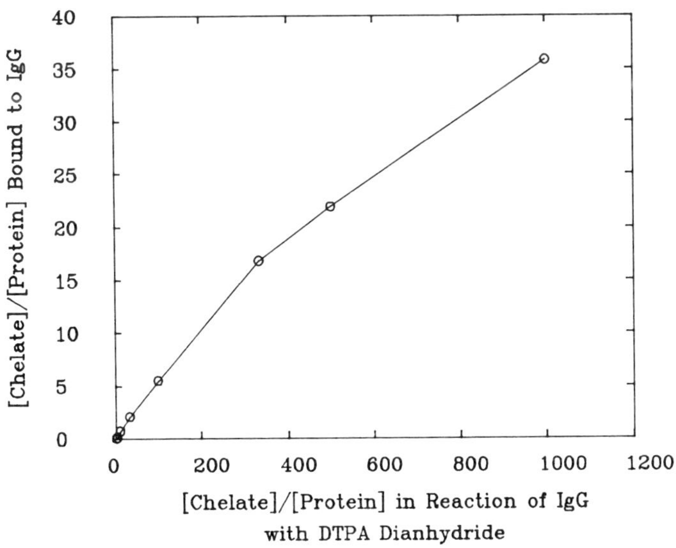

Figure 8. Concentration dependence of reaction of DTPA dianhydride with bovine IgG.

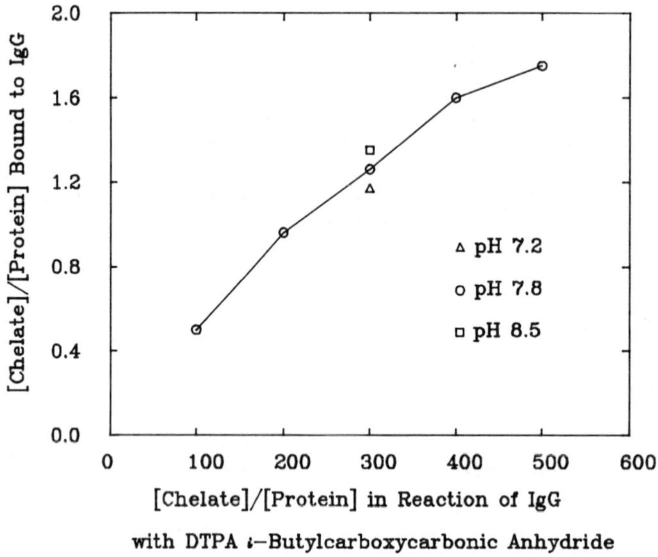

Figure 9. Concentration dependence of reaction of DTPA i-butylcarboxycarbonic anhydride with bovine IgG.

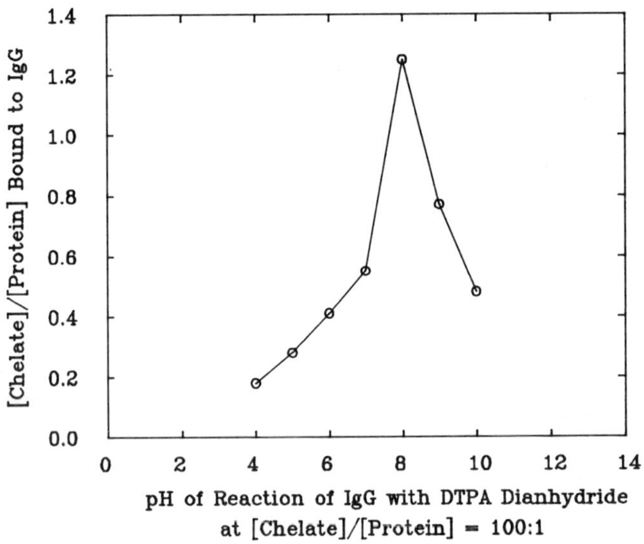

Figure 10. pH dependence of reaction of bovine IgG with DTPA dianhydride.

maximized at a solution pH near 8.0. This can be explained by an analysis of the chemistry of the conjugation. Reaction of the anhydride with ε amino groups of lysine will be favored by deprotonation in basic solution. Aqueous decomposition of the anhydrides is acid or base catalyzed, so it is not suprising that the conjugation reaction proceeds best under mildly basic conditions. Increasing anhydride concentration increases the number of ligands attached to immunoprotein. In addition, high numbers of attached ligands often adversely affect the specificity or reactivity of conjugated monoclonal antibodies.

The linking of a metal to an antibody could, in principle, be accomplished by forming the metal chelate either prior to or after attachment to protein. Success to date has been achieved only by formation of the protein-ligand conjugate before metal chelation. The complexation reaction has several general features. First, reactions between the metallic radionuclides and antibodies are almost always performed with sub-stoichiometric quantities of chelate and metal ion. It is therefore of the utmost importance that no carrier added metals obtained from commercial sources be exceedingly pure or else be purified prior to use. Reactions of "carrier added" metal solutions are not likely to be of use because of the ease with which available chelate sites become saturated. Because the formation of chelate complexes is usually a bimolecular reaction, the complexation will proceed optimally when more chelation sites are available. Similarly, the more isotope in solution, the faster the reaction. Employment of a carrier chelate to insure solubilization of the radiometal is of value to maximize available isotope and the acetate ion has proven useful.

Imaging and Therapy

Perhaps the greatest potential diagnostic use for radiolabeled monoclonal antibodies is tumor imaging. A number of radiohalides and radiometals have been suggested for this purpose (23). Antibody conjugated DTPA complexes have proven to be the most useful because of the variety of metals usable, the relative ease of protein conjugation, the retention of biological activity, and the stability of the conjugate *in vivo*. We have demonstrated that high resolution images of tumors can be obtained using radiometal chelate conjugated tumor specific antibody (3,4). Similar studies with I-131 labeled antibody did not produce usable scans (24). In recent gamma camera studies performed at the National Cancer Institute, indium-111 labelled specific antibody was also seen to provide images of solid human breast tumor tissues grown in athymic (nude) mice (25). Extension of these studies to human diagnosis is now underway.

Scheinberg and Strand (26) have addressed the therapeutic effects of a tumor-specific antibody against the Rauscher erythroleukemia. A dose response corrrelation between this antibody and tumor inhibition was measured. The dose response curve served then as a baseline for quantitation of the therapeutic effects of cytotoxic radionuclides conjugated to the antibody. Scheinberg and Strand reported that in this model system I-131 labeled antibodies are not more effective than the unlabeled antibody itself. This lack of therapeutic efficacy may result from the long range of the beta particles emitted, the long half-life of the nuclide as compared to the rapid catabolism of the cell bound antibody, or to the low density of radiation received by the tumor cells (20).

Potentially more cytotoxic are the α emitting radionuclides such as bismuth-212 which is obtained from a generator. This radiometal may be conjugated by antibodies derivatized with EDTA or DTPA ligands. The Bi-212 nuclide has a one hour half-life and emits α particles with a range of 40-90 microns. If Bi-212 had been substituted for In-111 in the leukemic tumor imaging experiments described above, several thousand rads of high LET radiation would have been delivered to the tumor, enough to insure total therapy.

The stability of bismuth DTPA chelates has been investigated *in vivo*. Both free bismuth and the complex were injected into normal and leukemic mice. As anticipated, the free metal was retained in substantial quantity in the liver and other organs, whereas the chelated metal cleared rapidly through the kidneys. Cell killing by Bi-212 labeled antibodies has been investigated *in vitro*. Therapeutic potency was high despite the low specific activity currently available (27). Experiments addressing the specificity, stability and therapeutic potency of Bi-212 antibody conjugates *in vivo* are in progress.

Acknowledgments

Research support from the National Cancer Institute, Grant NCI-NOICP81052 is acknowledged. Work at Argonne National Laboratory was performed under the auspices of the Office of Basic Energy Sciences, Division of Chemical Sciences, U.S. Department of Energy under contract W-31-109-ENG-38.

Literature Cited

1. G. Kohler and C. Milstein, *Nature (Lond.)*, 1975, *256*, 495.
2. D.M. Goldenberg, Ed., *Cancer Res.*, 40 (No.8), 1980, Part 2.
3. D.A. Scheinberg, M. Strand, and O.A. Gansow, in *Monoclonal Antibodies in Drug Development*, T.S. August, Ed., American Society for Pharmacology and Experimental Therapeutics, Bethesda, MD., 1981.
4. *Science*, 1982, *275*, 511.
5. S.E. Order, J.L. Klein, D.E. Hinger, P. Alderson, S. Siegelman, and P. Leichner, *Cancer Res.*, 1982, *42*, 44.
6. W.F. Bale, M.A. Contreras, and E.D. Grady, *ibid.*, 1980, *40*, 2965.

7. A.M. Friedman, M.R. Zalutsky, W. Wung and F. Buckingham, P.V. Harper, Jr., G.H. Scherr, R.W. Fitch, F.P. Stuart, and S.J. Simonian, Int. J. Nucl. Med. and Biol., 1977, 4, 219.
8. J. Smit, J. Myburgh and R.Neirinckx, Clin. Exp. Immunol., 1973, 14, 107.
9. W.D. Bloomer, W.H. McLaughlin, R.D. Neirinckx, S.J. Adelstein, P.R. Gordon, T.J. Ruth and A.P. Wolf, Science, 1981, 212, 340.
10. G.L. Zucchini and A.M. Friedman, Int. J. Nucl. Med. Biol., 1982, 9, 83.
11. M.K. Rosenow, G.L. Zucchini, D.M. Bridewell, F.D. Stuart, and A.M. Friedman, Int. J. Nucl. Med. Biol., in press.
12. F.P. Stuart, private communication.
13. A.M. Friedman, R. Atcher, and R. Seevers, to be published.
14. O.A. Gansow, R Kausar, and K.B. Triplett, J. Heterocyclic. Chem., 1981, 18, 297.
15. T. Peterson, Ph.D. thesis, Michigan State University, East Lansing, MI, 1982.
16. S.M. Yeh, D.G. Sherman and C.F. Meares, Anal. Biochem., 1979, 100, 152.
17. G.E. Krejcarek and K.L. Tucker, Biochem. Biophys. Res. Commun., 1977, 77, 581.
18. C. Paik, D.E. Herman, W.D. Eckelman and R.C. Reba, J. Radioanal. Chem., 1980, 57, 533.
19. J. Dazz, Switzerland Patent 17930, 1966. British Patent 1,161,461, 1967. U.S. Patent 3,660,388, 1972.
20. B.A. Khaw, J.T. Fallon, H.W. Strauss and E. Haber, Science, 1980, 209, 295.
21. Stability Constants of Metal-Ion Completes, Chemical Society Sp. Publ. Nos. 17, 25, Chemical Society, London, 1964, 1971. IUPAC Chemical Data Series, No. 22, Pergamon Press, New York, 1979.
22. D.J. Hnatowich, W.W. Layne and R.L. Childs, Int. J. Appl. Radiat. Isotopes., 1982, 33, 327.
23. D.A. Scheinberg, M. Strand and O.A. Gansow in Cell Fusion, E.G. Basset, Ed., Raven Press, 1983.
24. D.A. Scheinberg, W. Anderson, and M. Strand in Radioimmunoimaging, S. Burchiel and B. Rhodes, Eds., Elsevier, N.Y., 1982.
25. O.A. Gansow, D. Colcher, and J. Schlom, to be published.
26. D.A. Scheinberg and M. Strand, Cancer Res., 1982, 43 265.
27. M. Strand, D.A. Scheinberg, W. Anderson, O.A. Gansow and A.M. Friedman, Proceedings of the Armand Hammer Symposium, 1983, in press.

RECEIVED October 27, 1983

INDEXES

Author Index

Subject Index

W

X

Z

Production by Paula Bérard
Indexing by Deborah Corson
Jacket design by Anne G. Bigler

Elements typeset by Hot Type Ltd., Washington, DC
Printed and bound by Maple Press Co., York, PA

RECENT ACS BOOKS

"Polymer Adsorption and Dispersion Stability"
Edited by E. D. Goddard and B. Vincent
ACS SYMPOSIUM SERIES 240; 477 pp; ISBN 0-8412-0820-4

"Assessment and Management of Chemical Risks"
Edited by Joseph V. Rodricks and Robert C. Tardiff
ACS SYMPOSIUM SERIES 239; 192 pp; ISBN 0-8412-0821-2

"Chemical and Biological Controls in Forestry"
Edited by Willa Y. Garner and John Harvey, Jr.
ACS SYMPOSIUM SERIES 238; 406 pp; ISBN 0-8412-0818-2

"Chemical and Catalytic Reactor Modeling"
Edited by Milorad P. Dudukovic and Patrick L. Mills
ACS SYMPOSIUM SERIES 237; 240 pp; ISBN 0-8412-0815-8

"Multichannel Image Detectors Volume 2"
Edited by Yair Talmi
ACS SYMPOSIUM SERIES 236; 333 pp; ISBN 0-8412-0814-X

"Efficiency and Costing: Second Law Analysis of Processes"
Edited by Richard Gaggioli
ACS SYMPOSIUM SERIES 235; 262 pp; ISBN 0-8412-0811-5

"Xenobiotics in Foods and Feeds"
Edited by John W. Finley and Daniel E. Schwass
ACS SYMPOSIUM SERIES 234; 432 pp.; ISBN 0-8412-0809-3

"Nonlinear Optical Properties of Organic and Polymeric Materials"
Edited by David J. Williams
ACS SYMPOSIUM SERIES 233; 244 pp.; ISBN 0-8412-0802-6

"Rings, Clusters, and Polymers of the Main Group Elements"
Edited by Alan H. Cowley
ACS SYMPOSIUM SERIES 232; 182 pp.; ISBN 0-8412-0801-8

"Bacterial Lipopolysaccharides: Structure, Synthesis, and Activities"
Edited by Laurens Anderson and Frank M. Unger
ACS SYMPOSIUM SERIES 231; 326 pp.; ISBN 0-8412-0800-X

"Molecular-Based Study of Fluids"
Edited by J. M. Haile and G. A. Mansoori
ADVANCES IN CHEMISTRY 204; 524 pp.; ISBN 0-8412-0720-8

"Polymer Characterization--Spectroscopic,
Chromatographic and Physical Instrumental Methods"
Edited by Clara D. Craver
ADVANCES IN CHEMISTRY 203; 792 pp.; ISBN 0-8412-0700-3

THE SQUIBB INSTITUTE FOR MEDICAL RESEARCH
LIBRARY
SEP 14 1984
PRINCETON, N. J.

DISCARD